Contents

KT-166-667

Preface

This Pocket Consultant is intended to be a handbook of information on the medical management of patients with malignant disease, rather than a miniature textbook of cancer or a 'recipe-book' of chemotherapy regimes. The emphasis is, therefore, on the practical management of patients, the more common medical problems encountered and on the use of cytotoxic drugs.

An introductory chapter covers the basic principles of managing patients with cancer and this is followed by a discussion of the methods of assessing disease and response to treatment. A section on data collection and recording is included, because information omitted at the stage of patient assessment is often lost and this may have major repercussions, both for the patient and for any subsequent attempt to evaluate therapy.

Chapter 3 summarises the common management problems in patients with malignant disease. Some duplication is inevitable in this part of the book, as many problems encountered do not fit neatly under one heading and there is frequent cross-referencing. The drugs in common use are then discussed in Chapter 4, along with their toxicities, interactions and mode of administration. The Appendices comprise some commonly used chemotherapy regimes, nomograms, lists of further reading and useful addresses.

Acknowledgements

The authors would like to thank the following for permission to reproduce their work: Professor Sir Richard Doll and the *Journal of the Royal College of Physicians* for the figure on p. 5 (*J. Roy. Coll. Phys.* (1977) **11**, 125); the *Journal of the American Medical Association* for the figure on p. 6 (*JAMA* (1968) **203**, 34, copyright 1968 American Medical Association); the American Cancer Society for the figure on p. 7 reproduced from *Cancer Facts and Figures* (1980); Dr J.F.B. Stuart and Professor I.H. Stockley for permission to use their drug interaction chart on p. 158; Rhonda S. Yuille and the *British Medical Journal* for the table on drug handling on p. 162 (*Br. med. J.* (1981) **281**, 590); Ciba-Geigy Ltd, Basle, Switzerland for the body surface area nomogram on p. 188 reproduced from Documenta Geigy *Scientific Tables* 8th edition; Professor G.E. Mawer for the gentamicin nomogram on p. 189.

We would also like to thank D.E. Hands of the Wessex Regional Drug Information Centre and Miss P. Rose and staff of the Dietetic Department, Southampton General Hospital, for help and advice.

1.0 Introduction

1.0 Introduction

1.1 Epidemiology

Cancer is the second most common cause of death in Great Britain after coronary heart disease and there are approximately 10 000 cancer deaths in England and Wales each month. The 10 most common causes of death from cancer are shown in Fig. 1.1. It should be pointed out that where treatment has a significant effect on a tumour (e.g. testicular cancer or leukaemia), the prevalence of a disease will be much greater than indicated by mortality rates alone. Furthermore, such tumours will be much more commonly represented in a hospital population and have a proportionately greater amount of resources devoted to their care than the less responsive ones.

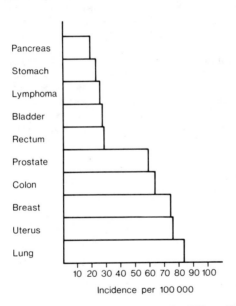

Fig. 1.1. *Age-adjusted tumour incidence rates for 1969 per 100 000 population in the USA.*

Over the past 50 years or so, dramatic changes have taken place in the management of malignant disease. In the past, little could be done if surgery failed to eradicate a tumour but, with the advances in surgical technique, the development of safe, effective, radio-therapy and the advent of a large range of cytotoxic drugs and hor-monal agents, the therapeutic alternatives are great and the overall

1.0 Introduction

1.1 Epidemiology

approach more aggressive. The skill of a modern oncologist (surgical, radiological and medical) is in applying the right treatment at the right time and in knowing when it is best *not* to treat at all.

Estimates of the overall cure rate for cancer vary from 25-41% in developed countries, depending on how and where the analysis was made. The types of tumours included or excluded (e.g. skin tumours), the accuracy of the data collection services, the extent of underdiagnosis (especially in elderly patients) and, most important of all, the definition of cure employed, will all affect the apparent 'cure' rate. The 5-year survival is the traditional indicator of curability and depends on the assumption that patients surviving for 5 years following the initial diagnosis are free of disease and unlikely to relapse subsequently. This will overestimate the incidence of 'cures', as some tumours continue to relapse up to 10 years or more after apparently successful treatment.

The incidence of, and deaths from, some tumours are falling, while those of others are rising (Figs. 1.2 and 1.3), presumably because of environmental factors. This makes the true impact of modern cancer treatment all the more difficult to assess. For some tumours, however, there is strong evidence that advances in treatment have had a truly beneficial effect on a defined population over the last 10 years.

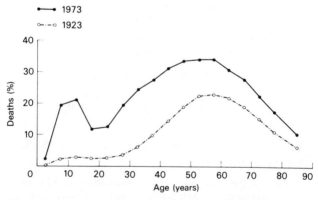

Fig. 1.2. *Percentage of all deaths attributed to cancer, by age, England and Wales, 1923 and 1973.*

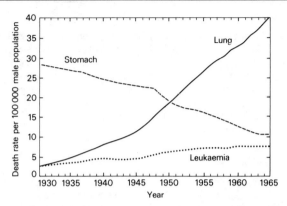

Fig. 1.3. *Cancer death rates by site in males between 1930 and 1965 in the USA.*

New therapeutic approaches are continually being evaluated in clinical trials. The most rigorous test of a new treatment is the randomised controlled trial but many studies continue to be published using matched historical controls or natural history data banks. The latter are much easier to obtain and the ethical problems involved in the execution of such studies are less formidable, although the conclusions derived are harder to substantiate.

In spite of widespread public and, indeed often medical, pessimism, life today for the cancer patient is of better quality than it was in the past and often lasts longer. Perhaps more important, there is evidence of improvement in prognosis for patients with some tumours, which should give hope to those who suffer from what is still the most feared of all diseases.

1.2 Principles of cancer management

Cancer is the collective term for a group of over 200 diseases, which have in common a growth-regulatory defect which enables the tumours to invade tissue locally and to disseminate throughout the body. It is not the intention of this book to describe the management of these individual tumours but there are certain fundamental principles that are essential to the good management of patients with cancer.

1.0 Introduction

1.2 Principles of cancer management

Diagnosis

It is important to confirm the diagnosis by histology or cytology (see section 2.2), not only to be sure that the patient does have a malignant tumour but also because precise histology may influence the choice of treatment and give a guide to prognosis. There are occasional situations where it is obvious that a patient has cancer, when biopsy may be difficult or hazardous and the result unlikely to influence treatment. These should, however, be uncommon exceptions to the rule.

Extent of disease

An attempt should be made to define the extent of disease or 'stage' the patient (see section 2.1). This should be based initially on clinical examination, blood tests and simple X-rays. In some situations, more invasive investigations, including laparotomy, may be justified but only if the results will influence the patient's eventual treatment.

Performance status

An assessment should be made of the patient's performance status or general fitness (see section 2.4), because this may reflect prognosis and influence the choice of treatment.

Treatment

When the basic information on diagnosis, stage and performance status is available, a clear decision should then be made as to whether to attempt to cure or palliate the patient's disease or to give symptomatic treatment alone.

Curative

Curative treatment is an attempt to destroy all malignant cells with one particular treatment or a combination of different ones. Such treatment must not only be directed at the primary tumour but also at all possible sites of local invasion or metastasis. For most solid tumours that are apparently localised, surgical excision is the treatment of choice and this may be followed by radiotherapy to the site of excision and/or adjuvant chemotherapy (see below). Curative treatment with radiotherapy is used when a localised tumour is surgically inoperable or when defined local spread may have occurred but disseminated metastases are unlikely (e.g. early stage II carcinoma of the cervix or Hodgkin's disease). When the tumour is widely disseminated (e.g. leukaemia or a solid tumour with multiple metastases), chemotherapy is the only method of attempting curative treatment (although it may be combined with radiotherapy and/or surgery). Although chemotherapy is only likely to result in long-term cures in a few very responsive tumours (e.g. teratoma, childhood leukaemia), applying the principles of curative treatment may prolong survival even if relapse eventually occurs.

Palliative

Palliative treatment is an attempt to relieve symptoms caused by a tumour, using specific antitumour therapy, with no intention and little expectation of cure. The symptoms should be carefully evaluated before and at regular intervals during, treatment and if there is no obvious response or unacceptable toxicity, treatment should be discontinued. Palliative chemotherapy should be given for at least 2 courses or 2 months, unless obvious progression occurs, if it is to have an adequate trial.

Symptomatic

Symptomatic treatment is the relief of symptoms using therapy with no direct antitumour effect. The most obvious example of this is the use of analgesics.

Adjuvant therapy

This is a term applied to chemotherapy given after local treatment, in tumours where dissemination is undetectable but can be assumed to have occurred. If effective, it should lead to a significant increase in the cure rate or overall disease-free survival. A theoretical advantage of adjuvant therapy is that treatment is given when the tumour volume is very small and apparently more sensitive to anticancer drugs. A number of points should be made about adjuvant therapy:

- its value has not yet been convincingly proved in any tumour
- long-term side-effects, such as sterility and secondary malignancy assume greater importance for younger patients or where prolonged survival can be anticipated (see section 4.4)
- morbidity and mortality from the short-term side-effects should ideally be low
- it can, at present, be recommended only in the context of clinical trials

---

Response

At the end of any course of treatment, an attempt should be made to assess the response (see section 2.5), by noting any change in performance status, symptoms and objective measurements of the tumour. This may necessitate repeating some or all of the initial staging investigations. The assessment of response should be clearly recorded before proceeding to further therapy.

Follow-up

Patients should be followed up regularly after treatment and follow-up continued indefinitely (though at increasingly longer intervals), even in patients remaining apparently disease-free. This is not only because of the risk of late relapse in some tumours (especially breast carcinoma and Hodgkin's disease) but, also, to check for any long-term toxicity (see section 4.4) and to record the patient's overall survival (see section 2.5).

Patient confidence

Cancer is a frightening disease for patients and the treatment is often complex and toxic. It is, therefore, very important to gain the patient's confidence and to allow time to explain everything clearly and answer questions as honestly and as fully as possible. This is particularly so at the start of treatment and whenever treatment is stopped or changed. Equally, it is essential to make sure that the patient's family practitioner is kept fully informed of diagnosis, prognosis, treatment and toxicity and also of what the patient has been told about his illness.

Terminology

The following terms are often used to describe the phases of chemotherapy and need definition.

Induction (or remission induction) treatment is the initial phase of intensive chemotherapy when an attempt is made to induce a complete remission (see section 2.5).

Consolidation treatment is chemotherapy given after achieving complete remission, in an attempt to make such a remission durable. It usually consists of the same intensive chemotherapy as remission induction, repeated for a limited number of courses.

1.2 Principles of cancer management

Maintenance treatment is given to maintain complete remission. It is usually less intensive and given less frequently but carried on for a prolonged period, perhaps up to 2 years.

Late intensification describes intensive chemotherapy, perhaps the same as used during the initial induction phase, given at the end of a prolonged period of complete remission and maintenance treatment.

Cranial prophylaxis is the use of cranial or craniospinal irradiation in combination with intrathecal chemotherapy, when complete remission has been achieved in tumours where there is a high likelihood of relapse within the central nervous system (CNS), e.g. lymphoblastic leukaemia and some lymphomas.

1.0 Introduction

Notes

1.0 Introduction

Notes

1.0 Introduction

Notes

2.0 Assessment

2.0 Assessment

2.1 Staging classifications

Staging is a measure of the extent of tumour in a particular patient. The purpose of it is to categorise the wide range of clinical presentations into groups with common prognoses and so dictate a suitable treatment policy. The principal distinction to be drawn is whether local, systemic or combined modality treatment is most appropriate. Staging can also be used to define accurately the extent of disease for trial stratification and, frequently, correlates well with prognosis. Staging may be either 'clinical' (essentially non-invasive) — based on clinical examination, together with biochemical, immunological and radiographic investigation — or pathological, based on histologically proven sites of disease. The latter is much more rigorous and where the result of an invasive staging procedure will not alter the management of a patient, it is not justified to subject that patient to the morbidity of the investigation. The financial cost of staging procedures can also be high and can be a major factor where resources are limited.

For most tumours, there is a simple system for classifying the extent of disease into three or four stages, which has practical use in deciding treatment and predicting prognosis. More complex and detailed classifications have been devised for many tumours, based on the tumour, nodes, metastases (TNM) system and depending often on accurate surgical and pathological information. For some tumours (e.g. breast and bladder carcinoma), the TNM staging does have some therapeutic and prognostic importance but for most, it is unnecessarily complicated.

Internationally agreed staging systems are useful for comparing results between centres but suffer from the drawback that they depend on how carefully staging investigations are done. The more sensitive the method of assessment, the more likely it is that a patient will be categorised as having an advanced stage which, in turn, may alter the treatment and affect trial analysis. Most staging classifications take no account of the prognostic importance of disease at a particular site or the risk of spread to further areas and may, therefore, incompletely reflect the bulk of tumour.

Breast carcinoma

The TNM classification of breast cancer is widely used and is shown below in full. A more recent introduction is the stage grouping (I–IV). A comparison of the two systems is shown in Table 2.1.

2.0 Assessment

2.1 Staging classifications

Table 2.1. Comparative classifications of breast carcinoma

Stage grouping	TNM system		
	Tumour	Nodes	Metastases
I	$T1_a$, $T1_b$	N0, $N1_a$	M0
II	$T1_a$, $T1_b$	$N1_b$	M0
	$T2_a$, $T2_b$	N0, $N1_a$	M0
	$T2_a$, $T2_b$	$N1_b$	M0
IIIa	$T3_a$, $T3_b$	N0, N1	M0
	$T1_{a,b}$, $T2_{a,b}$, $T3_{a,b}$	N2	M0
IIIb	$T1_{a,b}$, $T2_{a,b}$, $T3'_{a,b}$	N3	M0
	$T4_{a,b,c}$	Any N	M0
IV	Any T	Any N	M1

Pathological staging is very important, particularly in stage II (T1-2, N1-2 M0), where the prognosis depends on the number of histologically positive nodes.

TNM classification

T	Primary tumour
Tis	Pre-invasive carcinoma, intraduct carcinoma (non-infiltrating) or Paget's disease of the nipple
T0	No evidence of primary tumour
T1	Tumour <2 cm
$T1_a$	With no deep fixation to fascia or muscle
$T1_b$	With deep fixation
T2	Tumour >2 cm <5 cm
$T2_a$	With no deep fixation
$T2_b$	With deep fixation
T3	Tumour >5 cm
$T3_a$	With no deep fixation
$T3_b$	With deep fixation
T4	Tumour any size, with direct extension to chest wall (ribs, intercostal muscles, serratus anterior muscle) or skin
$T4_a$	With fixation to chest wall

2.0 Assessment

2.1 Staging classifications

T4$_b$	With skin infiltration (incl. 'peau d'orange' *or* ipsilateral satellite skin nodules)
T4$_c$	Both of above
TX	The minimum requirements to assess the primary tumour cannot be met

N	Regional lymph nodes
N0	No palpable ipsilateral axillary nodes
N1	Mobile ipsilateral axillary lymph nodes
N1$_a$	Nodes not considered malignant
N1$_b$	Nodes considered malignant
N2	Ipsilateral axillary nodes which are matted or fixed to other structures
N3	Ipsilateral supraclavicular or infraclavicular lymph nodes considered to be malignant or oedema of the arm
NX	The minimum requirements to assess the regional lymph nodes cannot be met

M	Distant metastases
M0	No evidence of distant metastases
M1	Evidence of distant metastases
MX	The minimum requirements to assess the presence of distant metastases cannot be met

The prefix p means post-surgical histopathological classification

Stage grouping

I	Disease confined to the breast with no fixation. <5 cm diameter
II	Spread to ipsilateral axillary node(s). No fixation. <5 cm diameter
III	Fixed ipsilateral axillary node(s) or deep or superficial tumour fixation or supraclavicular node metastases or primary size >5 cm diameter
IV	Distant spread

Chronic lymphocytic leukaemia

Stage 0 patients are diagnosed by chance. The degree of lymphocytosis in stage 0 is arbitrary but excludes reactive lymphocytosis, while maintaining the overlap with some forms of malignant lymphoma. The rate of progression is also an important prognostic feature.

0   Lymphocytosis ($> 15 \times 10^9/l$)

2.0 Assessment

2.1 Staging classifications

  Lymphocytes >40% of nucleated cells in bone marrow
I   As 0 but with enlarged lymph nodes
II As 0 but with enlarged spleen or liver or both; nodes may or
     may not be enlarged
III As 0, I or II but Hb concentration <11 g/dl
IV As 0, II or III but platelet count $< 100 \times 10^9$/dl
(Rai *et al.*, 1975)

Bladder carcinoma (American Joint Committee)

T_{is} Carcinoma *in situ*
T_a Papillary, non-invasive
T1   No extension beyond lamina propria
T2   No extension beyond half thickness of superficial muscle
T3   Invasion of deep muscle or perivesical tissue
T4   Invasion of prostate or other extravesical structures
N + Pelvic lymph node metastases
M + Metastatic disease other than nodes

Cervical carcinoma
(FIGO)

0   Carcinoma *in situ*
I   Confined to cervix
  Ia   Micro-invasive
  Ib   Invasive
II   Extension to vagina or parametrium
  IIa   Vagina (not lower third)
  IIb   Parametrium
III   Extension to lower vagina or pelvic wall
  IIIa Vagina (lower third)
  IIIb To pelvic side wall
IV   Further extension
  IVa Bladder/rectum beyond true pelvis
  IVb Distant organs

Colonic carcinoma

Various modifications have been proposed to the original Duke's classification shown below. These have subdivided the B category by depth of invasion and the C group by number of lymph nodes positive.

Duke's classification

A   Confined to the mucosa and submucosa

2.0 Assessment

2.1 Staging classifications

B   Spread through the muscularis
C   Spread to local lymph nodes
D   Distant metastases present

Head and neck tumours

It is impossible to include the various sites under one heading and the groups below should be used as a guide only. Reference should be made to the UICC manual on staging for the TNM classification.

I   Tumour confined to one site
II   Tumour involving two sites
III   Tumour with local infiltration and/or mobile ipsilateral nodes
IV   Extension to bone, muscle, skin, antrum and/or fixed or mobile nodes

Hodgkin's disease and lymphomas
(Ann Arbor classification)

The same classification is applied to both diseases, although in Hodgkin's disease spread is through contiguous node groups, usually from the neck through mediastinum, paraortic nodes and spleen, whereas in lymphomas it is much less predictable and the Ann Arbor classification is not very meaningful for them. Laparotomy is widely performed in early Hodgkin's (I-IIIa), which is the group for which local treatment is of value but it is not usually done in non-Hodgkin's lymphomas.

I   Single node region
II   Two or more node regions same side of diaphragm
III   Node regions both sides of diaphragm
IIIs   Spleen involvement
IV   Diffuse extranodal involvement
A   No symptoms
B   Weight loss (10%)/fever/sweating
E   Localised extranodal involvement
(Carbone *et al.*, 1971)

Nephroblastoma
(Wilms' tumour)

I   Tumour limited to the kidney and completely excised
II   Tumour extends beyond the kidney but is completely excised; includes spread to the para-aortic nodes, renal vein and pelvis
III   Incomplete excision, without haematogenous metastases
IV   Haematogenous metastases to lung, liver, bone, brain

2.0 Assessment

2.1 Staging classifications

V   Bilateral renal tumour
(D'Angio *et al.*, 1976)

Neuroblastoma

I   Tumour confined to organ or structure of origin
II   Tumour extends beyond the organ or structure of origin but
         not crossing the mid-line; ipsilateral lymph nodes may be
         involved
III   Tumour extends in continuity beyond the mid-line; bilateral
         regional lymph nodes may be involved
IV   Dissemination with metastases in the skeleton, soft tissues,
         liver, central nervous system
IV-S Otherwise as I or II with liver, spleen or bone marrow meta-
         stases but no radiological evidence of bone metastases
(Evans *et al.*, 1971)

Ovarian tumours (FIGO)

Ovarian carcinoma spreads insidiously throughout the pelvis and
peritoneum and the bulk of cases present as stage III. The prognosis
of stage Ic patients varies considerably as some of these cases have
widespread disease.

I   Limited to ovaries
 Ia   One ovary; no ascites
 Ib   Both ovaries; no ascites
 Ic   One or both ovaries, with cytologically positive ascites
II   With pelvic extension
 IIa   Uterus and/or tubes; no ascites
 IIb   Other pelvic tissues; no ascites
 IIc   Other pelvic tissues; with ascites
III   Extension to small bowel/omentum in true pelvis or intra-
         peritoneal metastases
IV   Spread outside the peritoneal cavity; pleural effusions must
         be confirmed as malignant by cytology; parenchymal liver
         involvement

Malignant melanoma

Prognosis in melanoma is best predicted by the measured depth of
invasion, together with the site of the primary, the trunk being
worse than the limbs. Clark's levels are shown for comparison.
Grouping by extent of metastases has little value, in view of the poor
response of this tumour to chemotherapy.

2.0 Assessment

2.1 Staging classifications

Clark's levels		Depth of invasion
I	Atypical melanocytic hyperplasia	
II	Tumour involving papillary dermis	<0.75 mm
III	Tumour extending to but not invading reticular dermis	0.75-1.5 mm
IV	Tumour invading reticular dermis	1.5-3.99 mm
V	Tumour invading subcutaneous tissue	>3.00 mm

Myeloma

Stage I — Low myeloma cell mass ($<0.6 \times 10^{12}m^2$)
  Criteria
  All of the following:
  Hb >10 g/dl
  Serum Ca^{2+} <3.0 mmol/l
  X-rays : normal bone structure or solitary lesion only
  M-component production rates:
    IgG <50 g/l
    IgA <30 g/l
    Urine light chain excretion <4 g/24 h

Stage II — Intermediate myeloma cell mass ($0.6-1.2 \times 10^{12}/m^2$)
  Criteria
  Fitting neither stage I nor III

Stage III — High myeloma: cell mass ($>1.2 \times 10^{12}$ cells/m²)
  Criteria
  Any of the following:
  Hb <8.5 g/dl
  Serum Ca^{2+} >3.0 mmol/l
  Advanced lytic bone lesions
  M-component production rates:
    IgG value >70 g/l
    IgA value >50 g/l
    Urine light chain excretion >4 g/24 h

Subclassified A or B, according to the absence or presence of renal impairment, respectively.
(Durie and Salmon, 1975)

Small-cell carcinoma of the bronchus

This is a rapidly growing disease and has frequently metastasised widely by the time of presentation. A complex TNM classification

2.0 Assessment

2.1 Staging classifications

has been described but is not very useful. The following simple classification is of greater practical and prognostic value:

Limited disease   Tumour confined to one hemithorax. Includes ipsilateral supraclavicular nodes but not where a pleural effusion is present

Extensive disease   Spread beyond the limits described above

Testicular tumours

There are 2 commonly used staging systems, both quoted below. The first is used widely in the USA, where retroperitoneal lymphadenectomy is routinely performed on early stage disease and so includes pathological information on these nodes. The second, Royal Marsden classification is more complex and detailed.

USA classification

I   Limited to testis alone
II   Testis and retroperitoneal nodes
III   Supradiaphragmatic involvement or extranodal extragonadal spread

(Einhorn *et al.*, 1977)

Royal Marsden classification

I   Lymphogram negative, no evidence of metastases
II   Lymphogram positive, metastases confined to abdominal nodes, 3 subgroups recognised
  IIa   maximum diameter of metastases <2 cm
  IIb   maximum diameter of metastases 2-5 cm
  IIc   maximum diameter of metastases > 5 cm
III   Involvement of supradiaphragmatic and infradiaphragmatic lymph nodes, no extralymphatic metastases
IV   Extralymphatic metastases. Suffixes: 0, lymphogram negative; a, b and c, as for stage II

Lung status
L1   <3 metastases
L2   multiple <2 cm maximum diameter
L3   multiple >2 cm diameter

Liver status
H +   liver involvement
(Peckham *et al.*, 1979)

Uterine carcinoma
(FIGO)

0	Carcinoma *in situ*
I	Confined to corpus
Ia	<8 cm cavity length
Ib	>8 cm cavity length
II	Extension to cervix
III	Extension beyond uterus in true pelvis
IV	Further extension
IVa	Bladder/rectum beyond true pelvis
IVb	Distant organ spread

2.2 Pathology

Accurate histological diagnosis is essential at an early stage in management. This requires an adequate tissue sample, although treatment can be based on a needle biopsy or cytology, if this is diagnostic. Where there is the slightest doubt, the interpretation should be discussed with the pathologist concerned and rare tumours, such as sarcomas, may have to be referred to the national tumour reference panels.

Other tests can contribute to the diagnosis and subtyping in some cases:

1. Pre- and post-operative alphafetoprotein (AFP) and human chorionic gonadotrophin (HCG) may help in the diagnosis of testicular tumours (see section 2.3).
2. Urinary vanilmandelic acid (VMA) in suspected neuroblastomas and carcinoid tumours (see section 2.3). Immunological markers performed on fresh tissue from a lymph node or bone marrow, give useful information in lymphomas and leukaemias.
3. Special stains and, more recently, immunocytochemistry, often provide useful information but may cause a delay in diagnosis.
4. Oestrogen and progesterone receptors are useful, some would say essential, in selecting the best management of patients with breast cancer; these require unfixed tissue.

Occasionally, a further biopsy is needed to clarify an area of doubt and, if so, care should be taken that the maximum information is obtained. The biopsy should be non-traumatised and fixed in small quantities, while keeping separate any samples required for frozen section or electron microscopy. Where a disease is thought to have transformed into a more malignant variant, e.g. in the nodular lymphomas, a repeat biopsy can be helpful.

For some tumours, histological grade correlates with survival (e.g. ovarian cancer) and can be used to assist in the selection of treatment. This has to be assessed by one observer to minimise variation.

In deciding on the relative benefits of local versus systemic treatment, knowledge of the routes of metastases can be useful. The pattern of metastases may also be of some help in deciding the likely source of disseminated tumour, where there is no obvious primary. The following lists are a guide but it should be remembered that any tumour *can* give rise to any pattern of metastases.

'Cannonball' pulmonary metastases

- thyroid
- testis
- kidney
- prostate
- melanoma

Bone metastases

- kidney
- lung
- breast
- prostate
- thyroid
- melanoma

CNS metastases

- lung
- breast
- lymphoma
- melanoma

2.3 Tumour markers

Biological markers of cancer may be derived from several sources:

- oncofetal antigens
- ectopic hormones

2.0 Assessment

2.3 Tumour markers

- enzymes
- products of tumour metabolism

Though tumour markers are being actively sought and extravagant claims have been made for their use, they can only be used to optimise treatment and make little impact on survival, unless effective therapy is available. They are useful in the following ways:

- to help establish the diagnosis of a particular tumour, e.g. the finding of a raised VMA helps confirm the diagnosis of neuro-blastoma
- to monitor response to therapy, e.g. β-HCG and AFP in teratomas
- to monitor for early relapse after a complete remission
- as a potential tool in the screening for cancer
- for the localisation of tumours by selective venous catheter-isation

The greatest problem in finding a useful tumour marker is the lack of specificity of most of the potential markers. Because of this, only a small number of markers are used clinically:

- Alpha-fetoprotein (AFP)
- carcinoembryonic antigen (CEA)
- β-human chorionic gonadotrophin (β-HCG)
- alkaline phosphatase
- acid phosphatase
- Vanilmandelic acid (VMA)
- immunoglobulin production in multiple myeloma and some lymphomas
- 5-hydroxyindole acetic acid (5-HIAA)

General principles for use

1. Always consider if there are other causes of a raised marker, apart from tumour.
2. If a tumour that commonly produces tumour markers (e.g. a testicular teratoma) is suspected, blood for levels of the usual markers should be taken *prior* to surgery.
3. After any treatment (surgical, radiotherapy or chemotherapy) in a patient with raised markers, *serial blood tests* for tumour markers should be taken to assess the response to that treatment. For some markers whose half-life is known (e.g. AFP and

27

β-HCG), it is possible to plot the expected fall of the marker, assuming that treatment has destroyed or removed all the tumour producing the marker (e.g. surgical removal of a testicular teratoma). Comparison of the actual rate of fall of the blood markers with the expected fall, will show if there is any remaining active tumour producing the marker. During prolonged treatments such as chemotherapy, *frequent markers* are obtained to ensure that the tumour is continuing to respond and the markers are falling.

4. After a complete remission (all tests normal including markers), follow-up marker studies can be used to detect relapse at an early stage.

Alpha-fetoprotein (AFP)

This is a serum protein which is present at high concentrations, prenatally. It is raised in malignant teratomas and in hepatocellular carcinoma. The half-life of AFP is about 6 days.

Non-malignant causes of a raised AFP include:

- viral hepatitis
- liver injuries causing hepatic regeneration
- inflammatory bowel disease
- during pregnancy (maternal and fetal blood)

Metastatic tumours in the liver, gall bladder carcinoma, prostatic carcinoma and lung cancer, are occasionally associated with a raised AFP.

β-human chorionic gonadotrophin (β-HCG)

With the introduction of radioimmunoassays, it has become possible to detect minute quantities of β-HCG. It is raised in choriocarcinomas and many teratomas. The half-life of β-HCG is about 30 hours.

β-HCG is raised in a number of non-malignant conditions:

- pregnancy
- testicular failure in men (there may be some cross-reaction of luteinising hormone (LH) with HCG in the assay)
- smokers of marijuana

β-HCG may also, occasionally, be raised in the presence of other tumours (liver, breast, stomach and ovary).

Carcinoembryonic antigen (CEA)

There used to be great hope for CEA as a tumour marker but this has not been fulfilled, mainly because of its lack of specificity. It is an oncofetal antigen and, in adults, was initially found in colon carcinoma, but it is also found in some patients with other tumours (breast, lung, pancreas, etc.).

CEA is found in a wide variety of non-malignant conditions, including:

- heavy smokers
- inflammatory bowel diseases
- hepatitis
- cirrhosis
- pancreatitis
- recent blood transfusion
- gastritis

The major roles of CEA are to monitor response to therapy, as a prognostic factor in colon cancer (raised levels at diagnosis indicate a worse outlook) and to detect early relapse. It is much less useful than β-HCG and AFP, partly because of its lack of specificity but, more importantly, because of the absence of effective treatments in the tumours in which it is found.

Alkaline phosphatase

Alkaline phosphatase derived from bone and liver, as well as ectopically synthesised placental alkaline phosphatase, can be used in the staging and monitoring of tumour response to therapy but, because elevation is very non-specific, its use is limited.

Acid phosphatase

This is raised in prostatic carcinoma and it is useful in diagnosis and monitoring of therapy. False-positives will result from haemolysis of blood samples.

2.0 Assessment

2.3 Tumour markers

Vanilmandelic acid (VMA)

VMA and homovanillic acid (HVA) are often elevated in neuro-blastoma. They can be useful in making the diagnosis and for monitoring treatment. A major problem with this test is the need for a special diet (eliminating foods such as chocolate, bananas and vanilla). However if VMA, HVA, total metanephrines, cystathione and creatinine are measured in a 24-hour urine collection, no dietary restriction is needed, though drugs containing catecholamines should be avoided.

Immunoglobulins and Bence-Jones protein (light chains)

Myeloma cells and the malignant lymphocytes of some lymphomas may produce idiotypic antibodies. This is useful for confirming the diagnosis, by finding monoclonal immunoglobulin in the serum or urine (light chains), in the case of myeloma and by finding surface or intracellular monoclonal antibody, in malignant lymphoma cells.

The response of multiple myeloma can be followed by monitoring the serum immunoglobulins. Lymphomas rarely produce large quantities of immunoglobulins which can be monitored in plasma but the presence or absence of cells producing monoclonal anti-bodies may improve our ability to detect small numbers of malignant cells.

5-hydroxyindole acetic acid (5-HIAA)

Carcinoid tumours produce large amounts of 5-HIAA. The presence of increased amounts in the urine helps to confirm the diagnosis. Serial urinary 5-HIAA levels can also be used to monitor the response of the tumour to treatment.

Other tumour-secreting hormones

A number of tumours may produce hormones (some ectopically) which can be used to help make a diagnosis or to monitor response to therapy. These include:

- medullary carcinoma of the thyroid (parathyroid hormone: PTH)
- lung cancer, especially small-cell (adrenocorticotrophic hormone (ACTH), antidiuretic hormone (ADH), melanocyte-stimulating hormone (MSH), thyroid-stimulating hormone (TSH), etc)
- pancreatic tumours (insulin, glucagon, gastrin)
- adrenal gland (ACTH, MSH)

- kidney (prolactin, PTH, renin, erythropoietin)
- rare ovarian tumours (17-ketosteroids)

2.4   Performance status

This arbitrary assessment of general well-being has been found to be remarkably useful in assessing prognosis and in the selection of patients suitable for intensive cytotoxic therapy. Many trials define a lower limit for inclusion in an attempt to limit morbidity and mortality attributable to non-malignant causes. Serial assessment by one observer also gives the most useful guide to progress and can be of help in making clinical decisions. Two scales are in common use and are described in Table 2.2. Undoubtedly, the correlation of performance status and results of cancer chemotherapy, depends on a number of interrelated factors such as age, stage, tumour bulk and extent of surgery if any, but in numerous studies it has emerged as an important prognostic variable, which is simple to use.

2.5   Response

Response is measurable change in the size of a tumour. It is frequently used as a guide to prognosis and it provides a convenient end-point at which to take clinical decisions. The following 4 categories are commonly used:

1. Complete remission: disappearance of all recognisable tumour masses and/or biochemical changes directly related to the tumour and resolution of symptoms.
2. Partial remission: >50% decrease in all tumour masses, measured by the product of the longest × the widest perpendicular diameters.
3. Progressive disease: occurrence of any new lesion or increase in the longest × widest perpendicular diameters of measurable disease of more than 33%.
4. Stable disease: changes smaller than those described above.

Response indicates sensitivity to therapy but may not necessarily equate with survival. The minimum duration of remission usually accepted is 4 weeks but it should be remembered that the biological significance of this depends on the rate of growth of the tumour. Certainly, the duration of remission or disease-free survival is a much better index of the effect of treatment. Good data of this sort

cont. on p. 34

Table 2.2. Two commonly used scales of performance status

Karnofsky scale		WHO performance scale (similar to ECOG)	
Scale	Performance	Scale	Performance
100	Normal, no complaints, no evidence of disease		
90	Able to carry on normal activity, minor signs or symptoms of disease	0	Able to carry out all normal activity without restriction
80	Normal activity with effort, some signs or symptoms of disease		
70	Cares for self, unable to carry on normal activity or do active work	1	Restricted in physically strenuous activity but ambulatory and able to carry out light work
60	Requires occasional assistance but is able to care for most of his needs	2	Ambulatory and capable of all self-care but unable to carry

Table 2.2. (cont.)

Karnofsky	Description		ECOG grade	ECOG description
				out any work; up and about more than 50% of waking hours
50	Requires considerable assistance and frequent medical care			
40	Disabled, requires special care and assistance			
			3	Capable of only limited self-care; confined to bed or chair more than 50% of waking hours
30	Severely disabled, hospitalisation is indicated, although death is not imminent	Unable to care for self, requires equivalent of institutional or hospital care; disease may be progressing rapidly		
			4	Completely disabled; cannot carry on any self-care; totally confined to bed or chair
20	Very sick, hospitalisation necessary, active supportive treatment necessary			
10	Moribund, fatal processes progressing rapidly			
0	Dead			

2.0 **Assessment**

2.5 Response

---

are difficult to obtain and few chemotherapy regimes have been assessed by the more rigorous criteria to date. Other end-points, such as increasing performance status or disease stabilisation, may be just as important in some patients. Like staging, the value of response to the patient depends largely on the sensitivity of the methods used to measure disease. For instance, response in testicular teratomas is a relatively defined end-point because of the sensitive biochemical markers that are available and the presence of metastatic disease in sites that can be well seen on X-rays. In contrast, ovarian cancer, where spread is characterised by insidious intra-abdominal growth, is difficult to assess by current imaging techniques. 'Second-look' surgery is undergoing evaluation as a possible solution to this problem but cannot at present be recommended as a routine procedure.

In general, there is only an increase in survival in patients who achieve a complete remission. A partial remission indicates significant drug activity and may be accompanied by a subjective improvement.

Survival, which is usually recorded as the time from diagnosis to death, is probably the best index of the efficacy of a particular treatment. But accurate survival data are often difficult to obtain (especially in tumours where there may be late relapses) and difficult to interpret, because allowance must be made for any subsequent treatment. This is particularly important where there is a very effective second-line treatment (e.g. chemotherapy for patients with Hodgkin's disease relapsing after radiotherapy).

2.6   Data collection

Chemotherapy records

It is essential that accurate details are recorded, preferably in duplicate, of all chemotherapy administered, e.g. in the patient's notes and on a separate record card or flow sheet. This applies to both oral and i.v. therapy and charts should incorporate an assessment of toxicity. A sample sheet where the toxicity is assessed on a modified WHO scale (Table 2.3) is shown in Fig. 2.1. The reason for a dose alteration or drug change should be clearly described, as it is almost impossible to assess retrospectively.

Patient records

Doctors are notoriously bad at keeping records of patient data and the standard hospital case record is more orientated towards a diagnostic work-up than close monitoring of complex therapy. However, much can be achieved by organising a simple system to collect and record some essential data. Exactly what information is recorded depends on the type of tumour, the availability of secretarial staff and whether the patient is part of a local or multicentre trial.

Frequent access to the patients' hospital notes is required to assess progress and check laboratory values. One advantage of laboratory values or X-rays is that the results are held on file at source and, if missing from the case notes, the information can be obtained retrospectively. Response is the most important clinical end-point to record because treatment is usually modified as a result. Simple clinical parameters that are an excellent guide to progress but often omitted are the patient's weight and performance status by one of the standard scales. Where a suitable marker is available, as in leukaemia (blast cell count), teratoma (AFP or HCG) and myeloma (immunoglobulin), it can be of great help in management to plot these on a chart showing the relationship to treatment cycles. Computerised systems are being introduced in certain centres but their consideration is outside the scope of this book.

2.0 Assessment

2.6 Data collection

MEDICAL ONCOLOGY UNIT Ht 1.9 m Wt 75 kg

NAME: FRANK N STEIN
HOSPITAL NO: 54321

			DATE:	1/4/82		22/4/82	
				Hb: 13.3		Hb: 12.0	
				WBC: 10.2		WBC: 4.8	
				Pls: 300		Pls: 250	
				WT: 75		WT: 75	
				SA: 2.0		SA: 2.0	
DRUG	Dose m²	ROUTE		COURSE NO.		COURSE NO.	
				Dose	Given	Dose	Given
CYCLOPHOSPHAMIDE	750mg	IV		1500	✓	1500	✓
ADRIAMYCIN	50mg	IV		100	✓	100	✓
VINCRISTINE	1·4mg	IV		2	✓	2	✓
PREDNISOLONE	100mg	O		200x	5	200x	5
			SIGNATURE	D.R. Acula		D.R. Acula	

TOXICITY

Karnofsky P.S.		7		8
Nausea & vomiting		0		2
Alopecia		0		1
Neuropathy		0		0
Mucositis		0		0
Cystitis		0		0

Fig. 2.1. *Chemotherapy prescription sheet and assessment of toxicity (continued on facing page).*

2.0 Assessment

2.6 Data collection

Surface area (SA) m² . 2 : 0 ..

13/5/82		/ /		/ /		/ /	
Hb: 12·0 WBC: 3·8 Pls: 200		Hb: WBC: Pls:		Hb: WBC: Pls:		Hb: WBC: Pls:	
WT: 75 SA:		WT: SA:		WT: SA:		WT: SA:	
COURSE NO. 2		COURSE NO.		COURSE NO.		COURSE NO.	
Dose	Given	Dose	Given	Dose	Given	Dose	Given
1500	✓						
100	✓						
2	✓						
200	× 5						
D.R.ACULA							

10							
2							
2							
1							
1							
0							

37

Table 2.3. Toxicity score.

	0	1	2	3	4
1 Haemorrhage	None	Petechiae	Mild blood loss	Gross blood loss	Debilitating blood loss
2 Oral	None	Soreness/erythema	Erythema, ulcers, can eat solids	Ulcers, requires liquid diet only	Feeding not possible
3 Nausea/vomiting	None	Nausea	Transient vomiting	Vomiting, requiring therapy	Intractable vomiting
4 Diarrhoea	None	Transient <2 days	Tolerable but >2 days	Intolerable, requiring therapy	Haemorrhagic dehydration
5 Constipation *	None	Mild	Moderate	Abdominal distension	Distension and vomiting
6 Bilirubin	<20	20-39	40-84	85-169	>170 μmol/l
7 AST	<50	50-99	100-199	200-399	>400 μ/l
8 ALT	<45	45-89	90-179	180-359	>360 μ/l
9 Alk. phos.	<340	340-699	700-1399	1400-2799	>2800 μ/l
10 Urea	<8.0	8.0-15.9	16.0-31.9	32.0-63.9	>64 mmol/l

		0	1	2	3	4
11	Serum creatinine	<150	150-299	300-399	600-1199	>1200 mmol/l
12	Proteinuria	None	1+, <3 g/l	2-3+, 3-10 g/l	4+, >10 g/l	Nephrotic syndrome
13	Cystitis	None	Mild frequency and dysuria	Severe frequency and dysuria	Frank haemorrhagic cystitis	Cystectomy needed
14	Sodium (low)	>130	129-120	119-110	109-100	<100 mmol/l
15	Calcium (low) (corrected for albumin)	>2.3	2.29-2.0	1.99-1.75	1.74-1.5	<1.5 mmol/l
16	Magnesium (low)	>0.70	0.69-0.60	0.59-0.40	0.30-0.20	<0.20 mmol/l
17	Pulmonary	None	Mild symptoms	Exertional dyspnoea	Dyspnoea at rest	Complete bed rest required
18	Fever-drug	None	Fever <38° C	Fever 38-40° C	Fever >40° C	Fever with hypotension
19	Allergic	None	Oedema	Bronchospasm, no parenteral therapy needed	Bronchospasm parenteral therapy required	Anaphylaxis
20	Cutaneous	None	Erythema	Dry desquamation, vesiculation, pruritus	Moist desquamation, ulceration	Exfoliative dermatitis necrosis requiring surgery
21	Rash	None	Mild (transient and/or localised)	Moderate (persistent and/or generalised)	Severe (confluent erythema)	Exfoliative dermatitis

Table 2.3. (cont.)

	0	1	2	3	4
22 Alopecia	None	Minimal hair loss	Moderate, patchy alopecia	Severe alopecia	Total alopecia
23 Infection (specify site)	None	Minor infection	Moderate infection	Major infection	Major infection with hypotension
24 Cardiac rhythm	Normal	Sinus tachycardia >110 at rest	Unifocal VE atrial arrhythmia	Multifocal VE	Ventricular tachycardia
25 Cardiac function	Normal	Asymptomatic, but abnormal cardiac sign	Transient symptomatic dysfunction, no therapy required	Symptomatic dysfunction, responsive to therapy	Symptomatic dysfunction, not responsive to therapy
26 Pericarditis	None	Asymptomatic effusion	Symptomatic, no tap required	Tamponade, tap required	Tamponade, surgery required
27 Raynaud's phenomenon	None	Occasional mild attacks	Frequent mild attacks	Frequent severe attacks	Gangrene
28 State of consciousness	Alert	Transient lethargy	Somnolence <50% of waking hours	Somnolent >50% of waking hours	Coma

29	Neuropathy	None	Paraesthesia and/or decreased tendon reflexes	Severe paraesthesia and/or mild weakness	Intolerable paraesthesia and/or marked motor loss	Paralysis
30	Ototoxicity	None	Difficulty with faint speech, soft transient tinnitus	Frequent difficulty with faint speech, soft persistent tinnitus	Frequent difficulty with loud speech, loud tinnitus	Hears only shouted/amplified speech, if at all; severe tinnitus
31	Pain **	None	Mild	Moderate	Severe	Intractable

* Constipation does not include constipation resulting from narcotics.   ** Treatment-related pain, not disease-related pain.

ALT Alananine aminotransferase.   AST Aspartate aminotransferase.

Alk. phos. Alkaline phosphatase.

2.0 Assessment

Notes

2.0 Assessment

Notes

2.0 Assessment

Notes

3.0 General management problems

3.0 General management problems

3.1 Metabolic problems

3.1 Metabolic problems

Acute renal failure

Although acute renal failure is most often seen in a setting of oliguria, it may occur without a fall in urinary output. The causes of acute renal failure in cancer patients fall into the following 4 major groups:

1. Tumour invasion. Extrarenal obstruction is common and caused by retroperitoneal nodes (lymphoma, testicular tumours), retroperitoneal tumour (sarcoma) and pelvic tumour (ovary, cervix, bladder, colon). Replacement of the renal parenchyma is uncommon, except in leukaemia or lymphoma.
2. Tumour products. Paraproteins are associated with multiple myeloma; the situation is made worse by dehydration. Uric acid is most commonly produced in leukaemias and lymphomas; prophylaxis should be given with allopurinol when rapid tumour lysis is expected.
3. Hypercalcaemia (see page 49).
4. Complications of therapy. These fall into 3 main groups:
   (a) Cytotoxic therapy. Complications with methotrexate are rare at normal doses; with streptozotocin, renal toxicity is dose-limiting and with cisplatin, complications can be minimised by an adequate hydration regime (see section 4.11).
   (b) Radiation nephritis.
   (c) Antimicrobial and fungal agents. Complications are caused by gentamicin (do not use with or after cisplatin), cephalosporins and amphotericin.

Management

As well as the general medical management of acute renal failure, specific measures may be required, depending on the underlying cause.

Extrarenal obstruction should always be considered as a cause of acute renal failure. Intravenous pyelogram (IVP), retrograde pyelography or abdominal ultrasound, are indicated if obstruction is suspected. Treatment will depend on the type of tumour causing the obstruction and sensitive tumours, such as lymphomas, may be treated with radiotherapy or chemotherapy. Unresponsive tumours may require bilateral ureteral diversion but, in the face of disseminated incurable cancer, a relatively pain-free death from uraemia may be preferable.

3.0 General management problems

3.1 Metabolic problems

Replacement of renal parenchyma by tumour is suggested by flank masses or enlarged renal outlines on X-ray and mild proteinuria, without nephrotic syndrome or hypertension, in patients with extensive lymphoma or leukaemia. Treatment is by chemotherapy but the outlook is generally poor, even if support is given by dialysis.

Renal failure caused by paraproteinaemia. A degree of renal insufficiency is very common in multiple myeloma though acute renal failure is uncommon. Dehydration is a common predisposing factor and is potentially reversible. Once renal failure has developed in these patients, the chances of a return to normal renal function are poor, despite chemotherapy and dialysis. Concomitant hypercalcaemia should be excluded.

Urate nephropathy is a complication most commonly found in acute leukaemia, Burkitt's lymphoma and other exquisitely chemosensitive tumours. The prevention and treatment of urate nephropathy caused by anticancer treatment is based on 3 principles:

1. Good hydration.
2. Allopurinol 300 mg/day orally to reduce the formation of uric acid.
3. Urinary alkalinisation to increase the solubility of uric acid. Once there is established renal failure with oliguria and rising urea, haemodialysis should be considered.

Methotrexate. When high doses of methotrexate are used with folinic acid rescue, the methotrexate may precipitate out in the kidneys. This may be prevented by vigorous hydration and urinary alkalinisation to increase methotrexate solubility (see section 4.10). Only patients with a normal creatinine clearance should receive high doses of methotrexate. If nephrotoxicity develops, methotrexate clearance is reduced and prolonged rescue is needed (methotrexate levels should be monitored).

Cisplatin. Prehydration (see section 4.11) with intravenous saline, with or without mannitol, diminishes the nephrotoxicity of cisplatin but renal impairment is still a problem with repeated treatment. Other potentially nephrotoxic drugs should never be used together with cisplatin.

Streptozotocin may cause a temporary rise in blood urea, proteinuria or severe tubule damage with Fanconi's syndrome. Stop the drug and watch for recovery. If the damage is mild and recovery rapid, the drug may be restarted.

3.0 General management problems

3.1 Metabolic problems

Radiation nephritis usually appears 6-12 months after completion of the radiotherapy and is characterised by malignant hypertension and acute renal failure. Death occurs in 50% of patients and chronic renal failure in the remainder. Nephritis of one kidney can also cause malignant hypertension. It should be avoided by careful radiation field-planning, with shielding of the kidneys or limiting of the dose to the renal beds.

Antimicrobial and fungal agents. Combinations of nephrotoxic drugs are best avoided and they should not be used with cisplatin.

Hypercalcaemia

Hypercalcaemia is a relatively common complication of advanced cancer and occurs both in solid tumours and in the haematological malignancies. It is most common in metastatic breast cancer (10-25% incidence). Remember that the calcium level must be corrected for the albumin and a normal total calcium may represent hypercalcaemia in a sick patient with hypoalbuminaemia. If unchecked, a vicious cycle of dehydration, prerenal and then intrinsic renal failure, will develop.

Symptoms

- lethargy and weakness, which may progress to stupor or coma
- loss of appetite, nausea and vomiting
- polyuria and dehydration
- constipation

Pathogenesis

- metastatic bone disease (especially from breast carcinoma, multiple myeloma and renal carcinoma). This may be mediated by prostaglandin production or secretion of 'osteoclast-activating factor' and can be exacerbated by immobilising the patient
- ectopic production of parathyroid hormone (especially in squamous-cell carcinoma of the bronchus)
- other causes: primary hyperparathyroidism, sarcoidosis, vitamin D excess

Treatment

This will depend on the calcium level and the condition of the patient. For mild elevations in an asymptomatic patient, oral hydration and treatment of the underlying tumour is all that is needed.

First line treatment involves the following measures:

1. Hydration. All symptomatic patients are dehydrated and prompt vigorous intravenous hydration is the single most important factor in the restoration of extracellular fluid volume and the glomerular filtration rate. Normal saline should be used as calcium excretion parallels sodium excretion.
2. Corticosteroids. Prednisolone at a dose of 40 mg/day will often reduce hypercalcaemia if used together with hydration and diuretics.
3. Diuretics. After rehydration, further calcium excretion can be accomplished with frusemide 40-80 mg every 6-8 hours.

Second line treatment is as follows:

1. Mithramycin (see section 3.2) inhibits osteoclast activity and is useful for resistant hypercalcaemia. The inhibition of bone reabsorption starts in about 6 hours and lasts 4-5 days. An injection of 25 μg/kg will often lower the calcium and may need to be repeated after 48 hours. It can be used chronically, every 3-7 days, at the risk of some toxicity but the main aim of treatment should be to control the underlying tumour.
2. Calcitonin rapidly inhibits bone absorption. The usual dose is 3-8 MRC units/kg, given as a 24 hours infusion (in a plastic bag).
3. Dialysis. This is capable of temporarily lowering the serum calcium level but should only be considered when renal function precludes forced diuresis and when the underlying cancer is treatable. It is rarely needed.
4. Indomethacin may be useful in patients with hypernephroma or squamous-cell carcinoma of the lung.
5. Inorganic phosphate (50 mmol in 1 litre, infused over 8 hours) can be used but may cause hypotension, renal failure or ectopic calcification.

Oral phosphate may be used for chronic treatment but causes diarrhoea.

Hypocalcaemia

Symptomatic hypocalcaemia is uncommon. The causes are:

3.0 General management problems

3.1 Metabolic problems

- parathyroid hormone deficiency: surgical ablation of parathyroid glands; destruction by tumour
- skeletal resistance to PTH: uraemia, magnesium deficiency, pseudohypoparathyroidism, vitamin K deficiency
- hypophosphataemia
- pancreatitis
- extensive osteoblastic activity (breast, prostate)
- chemotherapy agents: mithramycin, cisplatin (secondary to hypomagnesaemia)

Treatment consists of oral calcium supplements and, more rarely, i.v. calcium gluconate, in the acute situation and high-dose vitamin D or derivatives, for the long-term problem.

Hyponatraemia

The syndrome of inappropriate ADH secretion (SIADH) is a relatively common problem in cancer patients. It is characterised by hypo-osmolality, normovolaemia, normal renal and adrenal function, a less than maximally dilute urine and appreciable urinary sodium excretion.

Tumour-related causes include:

- carcinoma of the bronchus (especially small-cell)
- bronchial carcinoid
- adenocarcinoma of the pancreas
- carcinoma of the duodenum
- thymoma
- mesothelioma
- carcinoma of the larynx
- leukaemias
- Hodgkin's disease
- non-Hodgkin's lymphomas
- CNS metastases
- the anticancer drugs vincristine, cyclophosphamide

Treatment

1. The key to the treatment of SIADH is to treat and control the underlying tumour.
2. Fluid restriction (usually 1 litre/day) will restore osmolality towards normal.

3.0 General management problems

3.1 Metabolic problems

3. Hypertonic saline infusions have been advocated, as they result in a transient rise in serum sodium concentration but the volume expansion induces a rapid natriuresis and return of hypo-osmolarity.
4. Demeclocycline can partially inhibit the action of ADH (dose 0.6-1.2 g/day).

Hyperkalaemia

Hyperkalaemia may be life-threatening, causing depression of cardiac conduction, ventricular fibrillation or asystole, weakness, paralysis and ileus. In addition to the usual causes, it may result from very rapid tumour lysis (leukaemias and lymphomas). If a very chemosensitive tumour (e.g. Burkitt's lymphoma) is to be treated, the patient's electrocardiogram (ECG) and electrolytes should be monitored during the first hours of treatment. Therapy is designed to correct acidosis, quickly shift potassium into cells, increase potassium excretion and treat the underlying cause. The emergency treatment consists of:

- infusion of 50 ml of 50% dextrose i.v. with 10 units of soluble insulin
- infusion of 7 mmol (1 amp.) $CaCl_2$ i.v.
- infusion of 44 mmol (1 amp.) $NaHCO_3$ i.v. (more if severely acidotic)
- ion exchange resin (sodium polystyrene sulphonate by mouth or as an enema)
- monitor response by repeat ECG, potassium and HCO_3

Hypokalaemia

There are multiple causes of hypokalaemia, which is characterised by weakness and increased sensitivity of cardiac muscle to digoxin, cardiac arrhythmias, skeletal muscle and nervous tissue irritability and ileus. These include:

1. Alkalosis (respiratory or metabolic).
2. Excessive potassium loss in the urine, through diuretic drugs, syndromes of mineralocorticoid excess, renal tubular acidosis, magnesium deficiency, acute leukaemia, antibiotic therapy (especially carbenicillin).
3. Excessive potassium loss from the gastrointestinal tract, through diarrhoea, villous adenoma, laxative abuse, Zollinger-Ellison syndrome, medullary carcinoma of the thyroid, pancreatic cholera syndrome (vipoma).

Treatment

This depends on whether the hypokalaemia is caused by a total body deficit of potassium or a change in its distribution. In those with a depletion of the total body volume and metabolic alkalosis, treatment is the correction of hypovolaemia by infusion of normal saline. In those with increased total body volume but decreased effective circulating volume (hypo albuminaemia), colloid infusions may be needed. If sustained hypovolaemia has caused secondary hyperaldosteronism, potassium will need to be added. If a patient is in negative K^+ balance, replacement is necessary. Mild potassium deficiency can be corrected by liquid or slow K^+ but in severe symptomatic cases, i.v. administration may be necessary. Cellular uptake is not rapid and care must be taken to avoid hyperkalaemia. Generally, the infusion should not exceed 60-80 mmol/l and the infusion rate should not exceed 30-40 mmol/hour.

3.2 Infection in cancer patients

Prophylaxis

All cancer patients are at greater risk of developing infections of all kinds than are the healthy but those patients receiving intensive chemotherapy, causing prolonged neutropenia, are particularly vulnerable.

Strict avoidance of all possible sources of infection in the community is an unnecessary restriction for most patients on chemotherapy. During an epidemic of chicken-pox, however, particular care is advisable because of the risk of varicella-zoster, although in most cases the infectious period is past before a definite clinical diagnosis is made. Most bacterial infections are endogenous and arise from colonising organisms. The hospital environment is heavily contaminated with pathogens and infection may be transferred from staff, catheters, air, deposits of bacterial contamination in the ward and food, so a neutropenic patient who is otherwise well is probably safer at home, provided he can notify the hospital if he becomes unwell or develops a fever.

Precautions

• avoid urinary catheters if possible

- i.v. catheters: dress puncture site with antiseptic spray; avoid three-way taps and change site every 48-72 hours
- all invasive techniques must be aseptic

Gastrointestinal tract, vulval, vaginal and anal chemoprophylaxis, are not indicated routinely but may be applicable in acute leukaemia and for selected patients on chemotherapy for solid tumours. Oral co-trimoxazole and FRACON (appendix 1) are being used but no trial has conclusively proved their value. Both have side-effects and infections that do develop may be caused by resistant strains.

Isolation rooms are generally not necessary, except for specialised procedures such as marrow transplantation. Acute myeloid leukaemia patients undergoing intensive treatment for the induction of remission are often best nursed in hospital, because of the prolonged period of marrow depression and, if complete isolation is not possible, simple measures to prevent cross-infection from other patients (e.g. single room, washing hands before visiting the patient) are all that are needed.

Mouth care is of paramount importance in all patients receiving chemotherapy, especially when neutropenic, and they should be instructed to use regular antiseptic mouthwashes. The teeth should be cleaned with an electric toothbrush or cotton-wool-tipped swabs. If oral infection or ulceration develops, it should be treated rapidly and appropriately (see section 3.4).

Focal sepsis can be a problem, particularly on the skin and the area should be swabbed and an antibacterial cream applied. Frequent checks should be made for such pustules and, in particular, the perineal area should be examined regularly, as it is a common site of sepsis.

Immunisation

This is not available for any of the infections which commonly cause problems in immunosuppressed patients and, in those most at risk, the likelihood of an adequate immune response to the vaccine is low. Patients on cytotoxic chemotherapy or those with active lymphomas or haematological malignancies, should only be given vaccines of the killed type. A medical certificate of exemption should be given where a live type is requested for travel to certain parts of the world.

3.0   General management problems

3.2   Infection in cancer patients

Killed vaccines	Live vaccines
• polio (Salk)	• polio (Sabin)
• TB (BCG)	• measles
• influenza	• yellow fever
• typhoid	• smallpox
• paratyphoid	• rubella
• cholera	

Diagnosis of infection

While an accurate diagnosis is desirable, this should not delay starting treatment if the patient is neutropenic or becoming worse by the hour. As a guide, a temperature of 38°C, sustained for more than a few hours, is usually significant and, while it should be remembered that there are other causes of fever, e.g. the tumour itself (sarcoma, lymphoma), drugs (bleomycin) and blood transfusion, it is often safer to start treatment with antibiotics on the assumption of bacterial infection, once the relevant bacteriological specimens have been obtained.

Investigations

- one set of 3 blood-culture bottles (aerobic, anaerobic and fungal)
- swab ulcerated areas or areas of possible focal sepsis — send swab in transport medium
- screening swab — a throat swab is all that is required for detecting colonising hospital flora, e.g. *Pseudomonas aeruginosa*. Multiple swabbing from nose, ear, rectum and skin is not required
- midstream specimen of urine (MSU)
- full blood count (FBC) with neutrophil count
- chest X-ray
- 10 ml serum sample stored for later serological studies
- check for bleeding and give platelet and/or blood transfusion if required

Treatment of bacterial infections

Management is based on the 'best bet' hypothesis and should err on the side of overtreatment. The identity and sensitivity of known organisms should be used as a guide rather than as a mandate.

3.0 General management problems

3.2 Infection in cancer patients

Non-neutropenic patients (neutrophils $> 0.5 \times 10^9/l$)

A source of infection will usually be apparent and an appropriate antibiotic and route of administration selected. If there is no obvious source and treatment has to be started before cultures can be reported, an intravenous broad spectrum penicillin or cephalosporin may be given.

Neutropenic patients (neutrophils $< 0.5 \times 10^9/l$)

This group of patients can deteriorate with frightening rapidity to a seriously ill state and they may look and feel relatively well only minutes before circulatory collapse. It is, therefore, important to have a high index of suspicion and to act quickly if fever, unexplained hypotension or general deterioration occurs.

Gram-negative bacteraemia is a common cause of death in these patients and parenteral administration of high doses of two bactericidal antibiotics with a broad spectrum is standard treatment. Most have been based around an aminoglycoside (a) but this group should be avoided where cisplatin has been given in the preceding 28 days. Concern about the VIIIth nerve toxicity and renal failure has, however, led some physicians to favour the second or third generation cephalosporins (c). Their cost is higher but this is offset by the absence of drug monitoring costs. A broad spectrum penicillin with pseudomonas activity (b) is usually added. Table 3.1 shows the administration of different bactericidal antibiotics.

One antibiotic from each of groups a + b, b + c or a + c will provide a reasonable spectrum but consultation with the hospital bacteriologist is advised, because of local variations in organisms and their sensitivities. The cephalosporins and erythromycin have some activity against bacteroides but metronidazole can be added if these organisms are strongly suspected. Erythromycin is useful if penicillin sensitivity has been demonstrated or Legionnaire's disease is a possibility and cloxacillin if β-lactamase-producing staphylococcus is strongly suspected.

In the event of clinical improvement the minimum duration of antibiotic therapy should be 5 days, and treatment is often continued until the neutrophil count recovers.

If no response after 48-72 hours of parenteral antibiotics, take a further throat swab in Stuart's medium and a further set of blood cultures containing β-lactamase and reconsider the antibiotic policy

cont. on page 58

Table 3.1. Bactericidal antibiotics and their administration

Antibiotic	Dose per kg	Administration	
(a) Gentamicin	120 mg	8-hourly	Bolus*
(a) Amikacin	7.5 mg	12-hourly	Bolus
(b) Azlocillin	1.5 g	6-hourly	15 min infusion
(b) Carbenicillin	5 g	6-hourly	15 min infusion
(b) Piperacillin	4 g	6-hourly	30 min infusion
(b) Ticarcillin	5 g	8-hourly	15 min infusion
(c) Cefuroxime	1.5 g	8-hourly	Bolus ⎫ 50% dose reduction
(c) Cefoxitin	1.5 g	8-hourly	Bolus ⎬ for renal failure
(c) Cefotaxime	2 g	8-hourly	Bolus ⎭
Erythromycin	600 mg	6-hourly	60 min infusion
Cloxacillin	1 g	6-hourly	Bolus
Metronidazole	500 mg	8-hourly	15 min infusion

* Refer to Mawer's nomogram (appendix 3) for patients who weigh <70 kg or >80 kg or who have concomitant renal failure.

in the light of available laboratory reports.

If still no response to a second antibiotic combination after 5-7 days, consider non-bacterial cause for the fever.

Treatment of fungal infections

Antifungal therapy should be seriously considered if a high pyrexia persists for 7-10 days, in spite of adequate antimicrobial therapy and if cultures are repeatedly negative. The treatment is toxic, principally to the kidney. The optimum duration of treatment is controversial but is probably less than the 6-week period frequently quoted. Standard treatment is a combination of amphotericin and 5-fluorocytosine. Newer antifungals have been introduced in recent years and miconazole (i.v.) and ketoconazole (orally) have been successfully used in a number of mild and severe fungal infections, although significant hepatotoxicity has been recorded. Experience of their use in immunosuppressed patients is limited, however, and the combination of amphotericin and 5-fluorocytosine has not yet been improved on. The treatment should be administered as follows:

1. Take fungal blood cultures before starting therapy.
2. Amphotericin: start at 0.25 mg/kg per day by slow infusion over 6 hours, increasing to a standard dose of between 0.5 and 1.0 mg/kg per day. Monitor renal function.
3. 5-fluorocytosine: orally, 200 mg/kg per day in 4 divided doses; i.v., as orally but as a 20-40 min infusion. Reduce dose in renal failure.
4. Maintain therapy for at least a week after a normal temperature is achieved.

Oral candidiasis can progress to oesophageal candidiasis, which produces severe dysphagia and often pain. The diagnosis can be confirmed by endoscopy or barium swallow but these are seldom necessary.

Meningeal fungal infections with *Cryptococus neoformans* or *Candida albicans*, should be treated by systemic antifungal agents, as above. Intrathecal antifungal agents are rarely given but amphotericin B can be given by this route in severely ill patients.

Treatment of viral infections

Virus infections are probably more common in immunosuppressed patients than is realised and, undoubtedly, account for some febrile episodes that appear to respond to antibiotics and some that do not. Herpes virus infection is the most common clinical problem.

Treatment is as follows:

1. Take vesicle fluid or lesion swab into virus transport medium before starting therapy.
2. Herpes simplex oral and perioral lesions: give idoxuridine paint, 0.1%. Serious infections respond to acycloguanosine, 250 mg/m² i.v. 8-hourly.
3. Herpes zoster dermatomal lesions: idoxuridine 5% in DMSO, daily for 3 days. i.v. therapy is indicated only where there is evidence of dissemination. Early signs of this are satellite lesions or crossing of the mid-line by the rash. Vidarabine 10 mg/kg per day, for at least 5 days, has been used and acycloguanosine is a newer agent with encouraging reports to date.
4. Cytomegalovirus (CMV) presents with fever, malaise and, frequently, evidence of abnormal liver function. The diagnosis is confirmed in retrospect by a rising antibody titre but treatment is purely symptomatic.

Treatment of protozoal infections

These infections are rare but life-threatening and a high index of clinical suspicion is required. Cryptococcal meningitis and *Pneumocystis carinii* pneumonia are the 2 principal forms that affect cancer patients.

Cryptococcal meningitis

Headache may be present but fever and a gradually deteriorating mental state are common. Lumbar puncture is diagnostic and Indian ink preparations will demonstrate the yeast *Cryptococcus neoformans.* The treatment is i.v. antifungal therapy, as detailed above, with the addition of intrathecal amphotericin in severely ill patients.

Pneumocystis carinii

Rapidly progressive pulmonary shadows and dramatically increasing dyspnoea in a febrile patient characterise this infection. Patients with defects in cell-mediated immunity (e.g. Hodgkin's disease) are especially at risk. Diagnosis is best made by transbronchial lung biopsy if transtracheal aspiration has failed to show an organism.

Co-trimoxazole in high doses (4 tablets t.d.s.) has largely superseded pentamidine as the drug of choice.

Toxoplasma gondii

Severe disseminated infection, involving the heart, brain, liver and kidneys, can occur. The treatment is pyrimethamine, 25 mg daily, for 4 weeks.

3.3   Nutrition

Weight loss

This is a frequent problem in patients with malignant disease. It may occur as part of the advancing disease process or may result from the side-effects of treatment. Its causes are often multiple and ill-defined but it is very important to look for potentially reversible factors with careful history, examination and investigation.

Weight loss may be caused by one of the following:

- inadequate food intake
- malabsorption
- altered metabolism
- fluid loss

Inadequate food intake

This is the most important cause of weight loss and may result from one or more of the following:

1. Altered taste sensation: local effect of radiotherapy, chemo-therapy or, possibly, remote tumour effect.
2. Dry mouth: local effect of radiotherapy, chemotherapy, antihistamines, antidepressants.
3. Stomatitis (see section 3.4): local effect of radiotherapy, chemotherapy (especially adriamycin, bleomycin, methotrex-ate), monilia, herpes simplex, aphthous ulcers, iron and/or vitamin deficiency.
4. Dysphagia: mechanical obstruction from recurrent tumour, neuromuscular causes.
5. Oesophagitis: local effect of radiotherapy, chemotherapy (especially adriamycin, bleomycin and methotrexate), monilia, peptic causes.

3.0 General management problems

3.3 Nutrition

6. Dyspepsia: peptic ulcer (e.g. steroid-induced), oral chemotherapy, parenteral chemotherapy, tumour involvement in the stomach.
7. Anorexia: depression or, possibly, remote effect of tumour.
8. Nausea and vomiting: drugs (chemotherapy, opiates), hypercalcaemia (see section 3.1), uraemia, raised intracranial pressure (see section 3.8), intestinal obstruction (see section 3.4), ileus, abdominal radiotherapy.
9. Abdominal distension: ascites (see section 3.4), tumour mass, hepatomegaly, splenomegaly, intestinal obstruction (see section 3.4), constipation.

Malabsorption

This does not often contribute to weight loss in patients with malignancy but should be borne in mind and looked for, when clinically appropriate. Among the more important causes are:

- obstruction of the pancreatic duct (e.g. carcinoma of the pancreas, nodal metastases)
- obstruction of the common bile duct (carcinoma of the pancreas, nodes at porta hepatis, cholangiocarcinoma)
- coeliac disease (associated with small bowel lymphoma)
- lymphoma of the small bowel
- radiation
- fistula
- blind loop
- intestinal resection
- chemotherapy (fluorouracil (?), methotrexate)
- carcinoid syndrome
- VIPoma
- remote effect of tumour (?)

Altered metabolism

This seems to occur in a number of patients with malignant disease, quite apart from the effects of decreased food intake and malabsorption. Among the changes described are an increase in basal metabolic rate, glucose intolerance, increased lipolysis and negative nitrogen balance. The causes of these changes remain obscure but it has been suggested that some tumours release circulating factors analogous to hormones, which may produce these effects on metabolism and also, perhaps, induce anorexia and/or malabsorption.

3.0   General management problems

3.3   Nutrition

Nutritional assessment

Regular *weighing* is essential in the management of patients with
malignancy and provides a useful general assessment of nutritional
status *but* it should be remembered that changes in weight may be
caused by changes in fluid (e.g. oedema, ascites, pleural effusion)
and may not indicate changes in the body mass.

Muscle mass

This is a useful index and can be assessed by measuring triceps
skinfold thickness, with skin calipers and the arm circumference, at
the same level. The muscle circumference can then be derived from

muscle circumference $\simeq$ arm circumference $-$ skinfold thickness.

The mean muscle circumference in adults is 280 mm and a value less
than 200 mm suggests significant muscle wasting and less than
170 mm, severe wasting.

Laboratory tests

Tests of value in assessing nutritional status are:

- serum albumin
- serum transferrin
- thyroid-binding globulin
- 24-hour urea excretion

Nutritional support

A large number of patients will need either dietary advice or nutritional support during the course of the disease and treatment. There
is, at present, no good evidence in man to suggest that intensive
nutritional support increases tumour growth, enhances tumour
response to treatment or, directly, reverses the cachexia of
advanced malignancy. However, in general, a better nourished
patient is likely to have a higher performance status and be able to
tolerate more intensive treatment.

There are 3 ways in which nutritional support may be given:

- dietary advice and supplements
- enteral tube feeding
- parenteral (intravenous) nutrition

3.0 General management problems

3.3 Nutrition

Dietary advice and supplements

It is very useful to enlist the help of a qualified dietitian, who cannot only take an accurate dietary history but can also give detailed and specific advice to the patients, on problems such as constipation and dysphagia and can advise on the most appropriate supplements and feeds.

The most common dietary problems encountered in an oncology clinic are anorexia and nausea, associated with the disease or with therapy. They are difficult problems to deal with and, generally, only resolve when the tumour responds or when treatment is stopped. There are no convincingly effective anti-anorectic drugs but prednisolone 10-20 mg/day may sometimes be helpful. Anti-depressants may help if there is a true depressive component.

Some useful hints to anorectic patients include:

- eat little and often
- avoid the smell of cooking
- supplement meals with nourishing extras
- add extras (e.g. skimmed milk) to whatever is tolerated

A number of dietary supplements are available, some of which may be prescribed. Some serve purely as calorie supplements (e.g. Hycal) and some provide an appropriate balance of protein, carbohydrate, fat and vitamins and can be used as total diets. These supplements are usually made up to be taken as a drink. Unfortunately, patients often find them rather unpalatable, especially if there has been any change in the sense of taste because of disease or treatment. Osmotic diarrhoea may result if large quantities are taken at a time. Suggestions to make these supplements more palatable include the following:

- add acceptable food flavouring
- sip frequently rather than drink all at once
- chill before drinking
- sip through a straw from a covered container, if the smell is a problem

For further information, consult *Eating Well During Your Treatment* by R. de Pemberton (see appendix 7).

3.0 General management problems

3.3 Nutrition

Enteral tube feeding

Enteral tube feeding is a useful way of feeding patients who are unable to eat for themselves. It should, in general, only be considered when antitumour treatment, with a reasonable chance of cure or significant palliation, is being given at the same time. Once started in patients with advanced, intractable disease, it may be difficult to stop.

Indications are:

- mechanical obstruction to the upper gastrointestinal tract (e.g. carcinoma of the head and neck, oesophagus, stomach)
- severe stomatitis and/or oesophagitis
- severe anorexia

A number of *fine-bore nasogastric tube* systems are available, complete with bottles (or bags) and giving sets. It is preferable to use a system with reverse Luer locks, to prevent accidental i.v. infusion of enteral feeds. Fine-bore tubes are, usually, very well tolerated by the patient, compared with standard Ryles tubes.

Insertion does require care to ensure correct positioning of the tube. There is a possibility of insertion into the right main bronchus without producing significant discomfort to the patient. It is important to take the following steps:

1. Explain the procedure fully to the patient.
2. Ensure the introducer is in the tube and not protruding at the distal end.
3. Lubricate the tube with water or jelly.
4. Pass the tube through the nose and into the pharynx.
5. Encourage the patient to swallow and advance the tube slowly.
6. Do not force the tube down if the patient is coughing or choking —withdraw and start again.
7. When the tube is in the stomach, insufflate air with a 10 ml syringe (use 3-way tap if there is a reverse Luer lock on the tube) and auscultate over the epigastrium for bubbling.
8. If in any doubt, especially if the patient is uncomfortable, coughing or hoarse, check the position with chest X-ray.
9. Strap the proximal end of the tube to the patient's face or ear.

If there is partial oesophageal or gastric obstruction, the tube may be inserted under endoscopic control.

3.3 Nutrition

If there is complete mechanical obstruction, insertion of the tube through *gastrostomy* or *jejunostomy* should be considered.

There are a number of proprietary *feeds* available suitable for fine-bore tube feeding but feeds can also be prepared from components. The dietitian should be consulted for advice on the most appropriate feeds and regimes.

Unless there is evidence of intestinal malabsorption, feeds containing nitrogen as whole protein, rather than oligopeptides or free amino acids, are preferable. Although regimes should ideally be individualised for the patient, according to estimated calorie expenditure and nitrogen balance, for most adult patients who are not severely catabolic, a regime that provides 3 l of fluid, 2000-3000 Cal and about 10 g of nitrogen per day is satisfactory.

Feeds should ideally be given by continuous drip over 24 hours but, for a patient at home, feeds can be given as 4-6 aliquots, each run in over 2-3 hours. With this schedule, however, the incidence of gastrointestinal side-effects is likely to be greater and absorption less complete.

Vitamin supplements may need to be given with feeds.

The common complications of tube feeding are:

- tube blockage—fine-bore tubes need regular flushing with water
- tube regurgitation or accidental removal
- ulceration and stricture (rare with fine-bore tubes)
- introduction of tube into trachea
- diarrhoea
- abdominal pain, or bloating sensation
- hyperglycaemia
- hypokalaemia

Patients should be carefully monitored during feeding, with regular weighing, full blood count, urea and electrolytes and liver function tests.

In appropriate patients who have adequate support, enteral tube feeding can be managed at home.

3.0 General management problems

3.3 Nutrition

Parenteral nutrition

Parenteral nutrition should be considered in patients unable to tolerate enteral feeding. It should only be started in those thought to need temporary support during a crisis period, who have a reasonable chance of returning to normal feeding, because the treatment is complex, expensive and difficult to discontinue once started.

Patients in whom it should be considered include those with:

- severe treatment-related vomiting or enteritis
- intestinal obstruction by a treatable tumour
- extensive small-bowel lymphoma, with malabsorption or perforation
- small-bowel fistula

As with enteral tube feeding, there is no evidence that parenteral nutrition enhances tumour growth or response to therapy but it will improve the performance status of a cachetic patient and make him better able to tolerate treatment.

Parenteral nutrition must be given via a catheter in a large central vein, preferably the superior vena cava entered by subclavian vein catheterisation, because feeding solutions all tend to cause thrombosis if delivered via small peripheral veins. Scrupulous attention must be paid to aseptic technique, whenever the catheter is handled, because the risks of catheter-related infection are high, especially in immunosuppressed and neutropenic patients. All giving sets should be changed daily. As far as possible, drugs and blood should not be given through the same catheter as feeding solutions, but this may be unavoidable in patients with poor peripheral veins.

It is not appropriate to discuss here the details of parenteral nutrition and the relative merits of the solutions available. Regimes should, ideally, be designed for the individual patient and his metabolic requirements but a simple regime suitable for patients who are not very catabolic or in renal or hepatic failure, is shown in Table 3.2.

The more common complications of parenteral nutrition include:

- catheter-related infection
- fluid overload
- hyperglycaemia (give soluble insulin if necessary)

- electrolyte, trace metal and vitamin deficiencies
- disturbed liver function (elevated transaminases and alkaline phosphatase)

Patients receiving parenteral nutrition should be monitored with:

- temperature chart
- fluid balance chart
- daily weighing
- regular urea, electrolytes and glucose estimations (daily for first week)
- regular liver function tests
- urinalysis

Table 3.2. Intravenous feeding regime (for patients *not* severely catabolic and *not* in renal or hepatic failure). Administer via central venous catheter with Y connection

Time (hours)	Line 1	Line 2
08.00	Vamin Glucose 500 ml	Dextrose 20% 500 ml + 1 g KCl + 1 amp. Solivito
16.00	Vamin Glucose 500 ml	Intralipid 20% 500 ml + 1 amp. Vitlipid
24.00	Vamin Glucose 500 ml	Dextrose 20% 500 ml + 1 g KCl + 1 amp. Addamel

This gives: Volume 3 l,
Energy 11.4 mJ (2600 kcal)
Nitrogen 14.4 g

3.4 Gastrointestinal problems

Nausea and vomiting

This may be related to the presence of the cancer but the symptoms are more commonly encountered as a toxic effect of treatment.

3.0 General management problems

3.4 Gastrointestinal problems

Causes

1. Upper gastrointestinal tract tumours. In addition to the emetic effects, obstructive symptoms may be present and vomit may contain blood.
2. Small- or large-bowel obstruction. The cause may be intrinsic or extrinsic compression and other signs and symptoms of obstruction are usually present. The initial treatment is, usually, gastric aspiration and i.v. fluids.
3. Massive intra-abdominal tumour or tense ascites may cause nausea and vomiting by pressure effects on the stomach.
4. Metabolic causes, e.g. hypercalcaemia (see section 3.1), uraemia.
5. Opiate analgesics. Patients receiving regular anti-emetics may become tolerant of the emetic effect if the drug is continued. Tolerance does not develop to the analgesic effects. Nausea and vomiting can often be avoided by judicious choice of pain killers.
6. Raised intracranial pressure.
7. Radiotherapy often produces some nausea and occasional vomiting. Any large radiotherapy field will give malaise and nausea but large abdominal fields nearly always cause some nausea and vomiting. Anti-emetics are usually helpful.
8. Cytotoxic drugs. These are by far the most common cause of nausea and vomiting in cancer medicine. The problem is particularly severe with cisplatin, nitrogen mustard (mustine), nitrosoureas, dacarbazine (DTIC) and cyclophosphamide when given in high dose intravenously.
9. Ileus, which may be post-surgical or associated with vinca alkaloid use. The clinical picture is predominantly of the ileus and not the emesis.

Nausea and vomiting are common in many advanced tumours, even if there is no obvious biochemical or mechanical cause. These patients sometimes respond to steroids.

Anti-emetics

Recently, studies have tried to identify useful anti-emetics. Table 3.3 shows the commonly used drugs. No single anti-emetic regime is clearly superior and good control of the nausea and vomiting is not easily achieved. Most patients with mild-to-moderate nausea and vomiting benefit from treatment with a phenothiazine or metoclopramide but those with severe vomiting respond poorly. Patients

3.4 Gastrointestinal problems

Table 3.3. Anti-emetics commonly used to prevent nausea and vomiting in patients receiving cancer chemotherapy

Drugs	Usual dose
Prochlorperazine	5-10 mg orally, 4- to 8-hourly
	12.5 mg i.v.
	25 mg suppository, 4-hourly
Metoclopramide	10-20 mg orally, 3 hours before chemotherapy and then 3-hourly
	10 mg i.v. before chemotherapy and then orally, 3-hourly
Diazepam	0.07 mg/kg i.v. 30 min before chemotherapy and then 4-hourly
Haloperidol	1-2 mg orally, 8-hourly
Droperidol	0.5 mg i.v. repeated 4-hourly, increasing dose to 1.5 mg i.v. if tolerance develops
Nortriptyline } Fluphenazine	30 mg nortriptyline + 1.5 mg fluphenazine, 2 hours before chemotherapy
Triethylperazine	10 mg orally, 8-hourly
Dexamethasone	10 mg i.m. before chemotherapy
Chlorpromazine	25 mg i.m., 8-hourly

who do suffer nausea and vomiting after chemotherapy quickly become conditioned and will feel sick when, or even before, their treatment is given. This 'reflex' often includes the hospital environment so that they feel uncomfortable and nauseated on entering the chemotherapy department. Routine anti-emetics will not overcome this conditioning and it is, therefore, important to get the best anti-emetic control from the beginning.

It is important to remember that anti-emetic drugs may have unwanted side-effects, in particular drowsiness and extra-pyramidal syndromes.

Mouth ulceration

Apart from cancers of the mouth itself, ulceration of the mucous membranes is uncommon except when anticancer treatment has been used. There are several predisposing treatments and host-tissue factors, which make patients susceptible to oral ulceration but the main one is poor oral hygiene. Treatment-related factors include radiation and drug therapy.

General treatment

Prophylaxis is very important and all patients at risk should be taught to use regular antiseptic mouthwashes and brush their teeth regularly with a soft tooth-brush (electric if possible) or cotton-wool-tipped swabs. Mouthwashes should *not* contain alcohol.

Pain is a major problem, especially at meal times. Viscous lignocaine preparations (jelly or paste) can be used for temporary pain relief but they should be avoided when eating as they may interfere with the sensation of swallowing. Benzdyamine oral rinse is a new mouthwash that provides good pain relief and soluble aspirin gargles can be helpful.

Secondary bacterial infection may require treatment with an appropriate antibiotic. Gentian violet may also be useful and will dry the surface of the ulcers. Most patients, however, do not like the macabre effect produced by the violet staining.

In severe cases, vigorous cleaning and removal of exudate is necessary. If required, this should be done by a nurse after the patient has received an injection of opiate to reduce pain. Hydrogen peroxide mouthwashes are also useful for removing exudate, though they should be used sparingly.

If ulceration or a monilial infection develops, remove exudate before treatment and then give intensive antifungal agents. General care is of paramount importance. As soon as the drug-related neutropenia recovers, the monilia also usually improves.

Chemotherapy-induced oral ulceration

Anticancer drugs damage the rapidly dividing cells of the normal mucous membrane. Ulceration usually appears about 5 days after treatment and lasts 4-10 days. The severity of the effect can vary, from pain without loss of mucosal integrity, to total loss of the mucous membrane of the mouth. The condition can be further com-plicated by superinfection with monilia (see below). The drugs that most commonly cause mucous ulceration are:

- methotrexate
- 5-fluorouracil
- adriamycin
- bleomycin

Though mouthwashes of folinic acid may be useful in methotrexate-induced ulceration, no specific treatment is available and supportive care, plus good oral hygiene, is the only treatment available (see above).

Monilial ulceration is caused by a fungus which has a predilection for mucosal surfaces. It is a frequent contaminant of the skin and, when immunity is suppressed or mucous membranes are damaged, an oral infection is common. The appearance is of a white creamy exudate on an ulcerative base. This may be patchy or, in severe cases, involve nearly all the oropharynx. Infection of the oesophagus is quite common and this may cause retrosternal pain on swallowing. A barium swallow will show an appearance similar to that of oesophageal varices. Infection of the larynx is an unusual complication and, rarely, patients may develop a systemic infection.

Specific treatment comprises intensive use of antifungal agents:

- nystatin lozenges or suspension (100 000 units in 1 ml) 2- to 4-hourly
- amphotericin lozenges or suspension (100 mg in 1 ml) 4-hourly
- miconazole gel (5-10 ml) 6-hourly
- ketoconazole tablets 200 mg b.d. with meals

The lozenges should be held in the mouth, without sucking, for as long as possible, while the suspension can be swilled around the mouth and then swallowed.

Diarrhoea

This distressing symptom may be caused by the tumour itself, its treatment or, occasionally, by infections. Before starting treatment to relieve diarrhoea, it is important to be sure that the patient does not have faecal retention with overflow (do a P.R.) or incipient spinal cord compression (do a neurological examination).

If the diarrhoea is directly caused by the tumour, then specific anti-

3.4 Gastrointestinal problems

cancer treatment is of paramount importance. Diarrhoea is a common side-effect of pelvic radiotherapy and certain drugs but this can, usually, be controlled to allow treatment to continue. The common treatment-related causes of diarrhoea are as follows:

- anticancer drugs: 5-fluorouracil, methotrexate
- infection
- radiotherapy to the pelvis or whole abdomen
- broad-spectrum antibiotics

Specific treatment

- surgery, radiotherapy or chemotherapy, as indicated
- pancreatic enzyme replacements for the steatorrhoea caused by carcinoma of the pancreas
- methysergide (a serotonin antagonist) may be useful for controlling diarrhoea and malabsorption caused by a carcinoid tumour
- remember that the diarrhoea may be caused by tumour production of peptides

General treatment

The 2 most common antidiarrhoeal treatments are:

1. Codeine phosphate tablets 15-60 mg 3 times a day;
2. Diphenoxylate with atropine (Lomotil) 1-2 tablets, 4 times a day.

These drugs are usually effective alone but may be used together in severe cases.

Constipation

Many older patients with cancer complain of constipation. This may be a direct effect of the tumour or tumour-related hypercalcaemia, in which case antitumour therapy is of major importance. Narcotic analgesics are also a particular problem. The treatment of constipation, with the exception of an intestinal obstruction, is the judicious use of aperients. The 2 main types are:

1. Stool softeners: liquid paraffin, lactulose (Duphalac), methyl-cellulose and dioctyl sodium sulphosuccinate;
2. Purgatives: bisacodyl (Dulcolax), danthron (Dorbanex), senna (Senokot).

3.0 General management problems

3.4 Gastrointestinal problems

The most important drug-induced causes of constipation are the use of:

- strong analgesics
- vinca alkaloid drugs (these patients should be checked for constipation and treated early)

Most patients do best with a combination of both types of aperients and suggested regimes include:

- dioctyl sodium sulphonosuccinate tablets, 1-2 a day and senna 2-4 on alternate nights
- proprietary combined agents may also be used, such as Dorbanex Medo or Forte 5-10 ml, b.d. or t.d.s.

Patients who present with a loaded rectum and hard faeces often need an enema or bisacodyl suppository and, occasionally, a manual evacuation. Patients who, in spite of regular aperients, do not have their bowels open regularly, may need further suppositories every third day.

Ascites

Ascites is a frequent and troublesome problem in cancer patients. The common causes include:

- widespread tumour involvement of the peritoneum (especially in ovarian carcinoma, diffuse lymphoma), causing malignant ascites
- lymph node or tumour obstruction of the thoracic duct, causing characteristic chylous ('milky') ascites
- liver failure
- severe hypoalbuminaemia

Management

1. Confirm the diagnosis with liver function tests, serum albumin and diagnostic tap for cytology and bacteriology.
2. Symptomatic relief may be obtained by formal paracentesis (see below).
3. Diuretics (spironolactone ± frusemide) will help the ascites of liver failure and hypoalbuminaemia and, occasionally, malignant ascites.
4. Systemic chemotherapy is the treatment of choice for responsive tumours (e.g. lymphomas).

5. Intraperitoneal chemotherapy can be tried but is not usually very effective: bleomycin 30-90 mg or thiotepa 20-60 mg can be used (see section 4.15 for details of technique and complications).
6. Very viscid mucinous ascites (pseudomyxoma peritonei) cannot be drained but should be removed at laparotomy.

Paracentesis is a simple and relatively safe technique that can be repeated in patients with recurrent ascites. The following points are important to remember:

1. Confirm, by clinical examination, needle aspiration or ultrasound, that the abdominal swelling is caused by fluid, not massive tumour or intestinal obstruction.
2. A peritoneal dialysis catheter can be used and is more comfortable than trochar, cannula, and rubber catheter.
3. Insert catheter, preferably, in left iliac fossa but avoid obvious tumour masses or possible distended bowel.
4. Drain ascites slowly over 3-6 hours (rapid drainage may cause collapse and hypotension), positioning patient to get maximum drainage.
5. If significant amounts of fluid are still draining after 12-24 hours, remove catheter, because the rate of accumulation is obviously rapid and further drainage will only lead to hypovolaemia, hypoalbuminaemia and risks of infection.

Intestinal obstruction

This is a common presentation of colonic tumours and is often a feature of ovarian and other pelvic tumours, although it may also be caused by post-operative or post-radiotherapy adhesions. The management is always surgical, in the first instance, with removal of the tumour if possible or some form of bypass or stoma procedure, if not. This may be followed by chemotherapy or radiotherapy, in the rare instances of there being a responsive tumour.

Recurrent ovarian carcinoma presents particular problems, as the tumour is often widespread in the peritoneal cavity, with involvement of multiple loops of small and large bowel. This can cause an atypical and insidious presentation of subacute obstruction, sometimes with minimal signs and unusual radiological appearances. Because of the widespread involvement, surgery is not usually possible, although a surgical opinion should always be sought.

Chemotherapy offers some chance of palliation, but temporary relief can sometimes occur by a simple 'drip and suck' technique.

In patients with terminal disease and complete intestinal obstruction, a nasogastric tube may relieve the patient's vomiting but it is not very comfortable. With judicious use of anti-emetics and opiates, it should be possible to keep patients comfortable and vomiting to a minimum, for several days, without resort to nasogastric drainage.

3.5   Respiratory problems

Dyspnoea The most common symptom, and can be due to:

- anaemia
- anaphylaxis: bleomycin, asparaginase, cisplatin, etoposide, melphalan, blood products
- infection: viral, bacterial or protozoal
- pleural effusion
- lymphangitis
- bronchial obstruction
- drug-induced pneumonitis
- radiation-induced pneumonitis
- pain, e.g. rib fracture
- psychogenic causes
- other medical conditions: embolism, cardiac failure, asthma

Treatment depends on the underlying cause and many of the individual items are discussed below. It should be remembered that a chest X-ray may be normal, despite underlying bronchospasm, chronic bronchitis and emphysema, small metastases (< 6 mm), miliary TB, early interstitial pneumonia and acute pulmonary embolism. Severe dyspnoea in terminally ill patients is best relieved by opiates.

Chronic cough Due to metastases, can be suppressed with codeine linctus or a proprietary preparation, once infection has been excluded. The sputum should be examined, if possible and sent for culture, if appropriate.

Haemoptysis May either be due to primary tumour, pulmonary embolism or, rarely, metastases. It is not a common presentation of thrombocytopenia but since epistaxis is a much more frequent feature, there may be some confusion, as blood is often visible at the back of the pharynx. Chronic cough may produce a slightly blood-stained sputum. Loss of blood is rarely severe and episodes usually subside spontaneously, with sedation. Platelets may, however, be given if the peripheral count is less than $20 \times 10^9/l$. Urgent bronchoscopy should be considered if haemorrhage persists and there is no evidence of a coagulation disorder.

Stridor Can be caused by tumours of the thyroid, lung and oesophagus as well as the lymphomas and, usually, requires urgent radiotherapy to the area of obstruction. Prednisolone in high doses (40-60 mg daily) should be given, in addition, to reduce oedema and bronchospasm. If the tumour is very chemosensitive, e.g. lymphoma and the symptoms slight, chemotherapy can be used in the first instance and radiotherapy held in reserve.

Lymphangitis

This diffuse infiltration of the pulmonary lymphatics by tumour is usually bilateral and associated with progressive dyspnoea. It does not respond well to any measures and is usually associated with a poor prognosis. Specific cytotoxic chemotherapy is the treatment of choice and may improve survival in lymphomas and breast cancer. There are some reports of symptomatic relief by steroids.

Pleural effusions

These are common in patients with cancer and may present as dyspnoea, cough or pain. Infection and infarction are the common causes. The condition should be managed as follows:

1. Aspiration for diagnosis is essential and samples should be sent for culture and cytology.
2. Therapeutic aspiration should be performed if there is respiratory embarrassment.
3. Remove no more than 1500 ml at a single aspiration because of the risk of pulmonary oedema. Alternatively, a tube can be inserted and the pleural cavity drained to dryness at a rate of not more than 2 l in 12 hours.

The *treatment* of malignant effusions is straightforward but not always successful.

1. If the underlying tumour is chemosensitive, systemic treatment should be started without delay.
2. If the effusion is recurrent, instill intrapleural tetracycline 1 g or

bleomycin 30-90 mg in 100 ml saline, after aspiration to dryness (see section 4.15). Control is achieved in two-thirds of patients for up to 12 months. Fever and local pain can occur with both these treatments and hypotension with the latter.

3. Consider tube drainage in more chronic cases, applying continuous suction for up to 24-72 hours, with antibiotic cover.

Pulmonary embolism

Pulmonary embolism is a common cause of death in patients with cancer. Gastric and pancreatic cancers have a particularly high incidence but other solid tumours also show an association and debility and immobilisation may exacerbate the problem. Frequently, the clinical picture, an ECG and chest X-ray, may be sufficient for treatment to be started. This should be as follows:

- heparin 1000 units/hour i.v., given for 2-5 days
- haemorrhage can be quickly reversed during this time by protamine sulphate
- warfarinisation can be started and the heparin discontinued, once prothrombin time control is achieved

Age and thrombocytopenia are frequent relative contraindications to anticoagulation in cancer patients.

Radiation pneumonitis

This commonly presents as dyspnoea, coming on 2-6 months after radiotherapy. The incidence depends on the dose, dose rate and volume of lung irradiated. Other factors include the following:

- adriamycin and actinomycin enhance the *radiation* damage if given before or with the radiotherapy
- sudden withdrawal of high-dose steroid therapy can reactivate latent lung damage
- concomitant bleomycin and radiation enhances the *drug* damage

The clinical features are:

- dyspnoea
- fever
- cough
- 'fluffy' shadows on chest X-ray

3.0   General management problems

3.5   Respiratory problems

The main problem is distinguishing pneumonitis from underlying
infection or tumour progression. The symptoms resolve with time
but the radiographic abnormalities persist. If bronchospasm is the
principal problem, steroid therapy may be indicated — prednisolone
40 mg daily until symptoms improve, followed by gradual reduction.

Drug-induced pneumonitis

Almost all cytotoxic drugs can produce a pneumonitis, which
usually presents as diffuse infiltration of both lung fields on chest
X-ray. Bleomycin and busulphan are the 2 most common causative
agents and give rise to a progressive interstitial shadowing and a
severe restrictive ventilatory defect. Methotrexate may give a fine
reticular shadowing but rarely are the symptoms severe. High-dose
oxygen is thought to exacerbate the toxicity of bleomycin and the
anaesthetist should be advised accordingly if a general anaesthetic
is being contemplated in a patient receiving this agent. Significant
reversal is seldom possible and management consists of:

- stopping the drug as soon as the diagnosis is considered likely
- prednisolone 40 mg daily

Tuberculosis

Reactivation of TB is possible in all patients with malignant disease,
and should always be borne in mind where there is immuno-
suppression. It should be considered in the following situations:

- prolonged pyrexia of unknown origin
- lack of response to antibiotics
- pancytopenia
- alcoholism or diabetes mellitus
- the elderly

The standard treatment in the established case is rifampicin 600 mg
daily, + isoniazid 300 mg daily, + ethambutol 15 mg/kg per day for
a period of at least 9 months.

In some high-risk patients, such as those previously treated for TB
or with old tuberculous lesions on chest X-ray, who are receiving
chemotherapy or high-dose steroids, prophylactic treatment with
rifampicin and isoniazid for 3-6 months should be considered.

Diffuse infiltrative shadows on a chest X-ray

A full discussion of the difficult problem of differential diagnosis will be found in a standard textbook of medicine. The urgency of diagnosis depends on the condition of the patient and the rate of progression. In the immunosuppressed patient who is deteriorating, the sputum and blood may be cultured. The most helpful investigations are, however, transtracheal aspiration and transbronchial lung biopsy. Close consultation with the bacteriology department is required to ensure that the specimens are processed correctly. Different causes are listed below:

- infections: viral (cytomegalovirus, measles, varicella zoster), bacterial (TB, coliforms, legionnaire's, rickettsia), fungal (aspergillosis), parasitic (*Pneumocystis carinii*)
- drugs: bleomycin, busulphan, cyclophosphamide, methotrexate
- metabolic: uraemia
- physical: irradiation
- circulatory: multiple pulmonary emboli
- neoplastic: lymphangitis, histiocytosis X
- immunologic: type III responses (e.g. farmer's lung), collagen disorders (polyarteritis nodosa, Wegener's granulomatosis, sarcoidosis)

3.6 Cardiovascular problems

Heart failure

Many patients with malignant disease are middle-aged and elderly and have a high incidence of overt or asymptomatic ischaemic and degenerative heart disease. They are, therefore, at risk of developing heart failure. The most common precipitating factors are:

- anaemia, caused by marrow depression from drugs or metastases, gastrointestinal bleeding, haematuria, haemolysis
- fluid overload during chemotherapy, e.g. hydration during cisplatin administration
- fluid retention due to corticosteroids, oestrogens
- cardiomyopathy: drug-induced (adriamycin, daunorubicin, high-dose cyclophosphamide)
- dysrhythmias (see below)
- tumour infiltration of the myocardium, especially in bronchial and breast carcinoma, and mediastinal tumours
- renal failure: drug-induced (cisplatin, methotrexate)

3.6 Cardiovascular problems

Management is the conventional treatment of heart failure and, where possible, of the underlying cause.

Dysrhythmia

As with heart failure, the more elderly patients are at risk because of underlying ischaemic and degenerative heart disease. Dysrhythmia in cancer patients may, however, be precipitated by:

- drugs (adriamycin, daunorubicin, high-dose fluorouracil)
- tumour infiltration of the myocardium, especially bronchial and breast carcinoma, lymphoma

Treat the dysrhythmia conventionally according to ECG findings and treat the underlying cause, if possible.

Superior vena cava (SVC) obstruction

This is a common oncological emergency. It should be looked for carefully in patients at risk, recognized early if possible and treated urgently. The tumours most commonly causing obstruction are:

- bronchial carcinoma (especially right-sided tumours)
- lymphoma
- Hodgkin's disease
- teratoma

Early SVC obstruction is often misdiagnosed as heart failure. The clinical features are:

- increasing dyspnoea
- headache
- swelling of hands neck and face, especially in the mornings
- fixed elevation of JVP
- suffused conjunctivae
- papilloedema and retinal venous engorgement
- sometimes associated with stridor

Treatment is urgent and consists of:

- dexamethasone 4 mg q.d.s.
- radiotherapy
- chemotherapy, if there is a likelihood of rapid response, e.g. in diffuse lymphoma, small-cell carcinoma of the bronchus. *Do not* inject drugs into arm veins if they do not collapse on arm raising

- oxygen—useful in high concentration if there is associated stridor

There may be persistent signs after treatment, since thrombosis of the SVC may never resolve or recanalise

Recurrent SVC obstruction following radiotherapy and chemo-therapy is difficult to treat and is associated with a poor prognosis. Consider opiates if symptoms are distressing.

Pericardial effusion and tamponade

Pericardial effusion leading to cardiac tamponade can occasionally occur in patients with malignant disease. The most usual cause is direct tumour involvement of the pericardium, with a reactive effusion. The tumours most likely to cause pericardial effusion are:

- bronchial carcinoma
- breast carcinoma
- lymphoma
- acute leukaemia

Clinical features

- increasing dyspnoea
- precordial pain
- dizziness
- tachycardia
- elevated JVP
- 'low cardiac output' state
- pulsus paradoxus—exaggeration of normal decrease in pulse pressure on inspiration (a useful, but not necessarily diagnostic, sign)
- soft heart sounds ± pericardial friction rub
- enlarged globular heart shadow on chest X-ray

Diagnosis

This should be confirmed by echocardiography.

Management

This is urgent and consists of:

- aspiration of the pericardial sac with appropriate cytological and bacteriological investigation

3.6   Cardiovascular problems

- radiotherapy
- chemotherapy, if a rapid response is likely (e.g. small-cell carcinoma of the bronchus, lymphoma)
- intracavitary drugs (see section 4.15)
- pericardial 'window' surgical drainage if the condition is a persistent or recurrent problem

Thrombotic problems

Patients with malignant disease have an increased incidence of venous thrombosis, both deep and superficial. This may, in part, be due to a remote effect of the tumour (e.g. Trousseau's syndrome — flitting thrombophlebitis as a marker of otherwise occult internal malignancy, especially of gastrointestinal origin; see section 3.7).

Other causes of venous thrombosis in patients with cancer include:

- retroperitoneal tumour
- pelvic tumour
- lymphadenopathy, especially iliac, inguinal and femoral
- oestrogens
- operation
- immobility
- i.v. chemotherapy — *never* use foot or leg veins (see section 4.6)

Management

This is conventional with analgesics (if necessary), support bandaging and elevation. The decision as to whether to give anticoagulants is often difficult and an assessment must be made of the potential benefits (prevention of pulmonary embolus), against the hazards of haemorrhage and the difficulties of anticoagulant control in patients on complex and, perhaps, intermittent drug therapy.

Anticoagulation is strongly contraindicated in most patients who are, or who are likely to be, thrombocytopenic. It also seems inappropriate to burden patients, who have terminal malignancy and venous thrombosis, with the added complications of anticoagulant therapy.

Pulmonary embolus (see section 3.5)

Once one pulmonary embolus has occurred, the risk of a subsequent and possibly more serious embolus is high. This risk has to be carefully weighed against that of potentially fatal haemorrhage from the complications of anticoagulant therapy. Many of the cytotoxic drugs, analgesics and sedatives used in cancer patients are protein-bound and interact with oral anticoagulants. Heparin has a much more rapid onset and can be quickly reversed by protamine.

3.7   Haematological problems

These problems, caused by the underlying tumour or its treatment, are common in cancer patients.

Bone marrow failure in cancer patients may, in general, be caused by 2 distinct processes:

1.   Bone marrow depression due to cytotoxic drugs, radiotherapy or other toxins.
2.   Bone marrow infiltration by tumour cells.

The complications of both are similar, as is the supportive care, but the treatment of the underlying cause is often quite different. Separation of the 2 processes depends on a number of factors:

1.   The presence of known tumour in the bone marrow, although sampling error can give a false-negative result on aspirate or trephine.
2.   The time-scale of the fall in the formed elements.
3.   The relationship of the change in haemoglobin, white-cell count and platelets to cycles of chemotherapy.

Bone marrow depression

The white blood cell count falls first, generally in 5-10 days, followed by the platelet count at 10-14 days and the haemoglobin at a much slower rate, owing to the long red blood cell survival. Some drugs, e.g. the nitrosoureas, cause a more prolonged suppression of the bone marrow, with neutropenia and thrombocytopenia lasting weeks or months. Slow release of methotrexate from a reservoir site, such as an effusion or the cerebrospinal fluid (CSF) can also give a similar effect, although this can be reversed to some extent by folinic acid (see sections 4.2 and 4.6). After prolonged chemotherapy, marrow reserve is depleted and a given dose of drug(s) will produce a greater degree of suppression. Rarely, a hypoplastic or aplastic state develops and may herald a secondary leukaemic process.

Bone marrow infiltration

This may be present from the start or develop during the course of disease, in which case thrombocytopenia is usually the presenting feature. Quantification of the degree of infiltration is rarely possible, except in the leukaemias but, in the case of the lymphomas, a qualitative assessment can often be made of the response to therapy. Solid tumour marrow infiltration is a poor prognostic sign and rarely indicates curability.

Where infiltration is present, chemotherapy is the only modality likely to be effective. As pancytopenia of variable degree is often present, the usual guidelines for dose reduction based on white blood cell and platelet count do not apply. It is common practice to start with about 75% of calculated cytotoxic drug doses, observe the haematologic indices carefully and be ready to support the patient actively, if necessary. The indices should improve eventually if effective treatment is being given but, often, a mixed picture of failure and depression is present and, in these cases, charting the haemoglobin, white blood cell count and platelets, together with the chemotherapy given, can greatly assist management.

Anaemia

This is a common presenting feature of cancer and arises through a variety of causes:

- blood loss — iron deficiency anaemia
- infection
- metastatic involvement of the bone marrow
- disturbance of nutrition
- acquired haemolytic anaemia
- impaired renal function
- bone marrow depression because of treatment
- anaemia of disseminated malignancy

Blood loss

This results in an iron-deficiency anaemia and, as shown in Table 3.4, certain tumours are an important cause of this type of anaemia. The findings on a blood film are of a hypochromic microcytic anaemia. The reticulocyte count is usually normal but may be slightly raised (2-5%), if there has been recent haemorrhage. Serum iron is reduced and the total iron-binding capacity of the serum is

Table 3.4. Common causes of iron-deficiency anaemia

Women in reproductive life
  Menstruation
  Pregnancy
  Poor diet
  Childbirth

Men and women (general)
  Peptic ulcer
  Hiatus hernia
  Haemorrhoids
  Gastrointestinal tract tumours (oesophagus, stomach, colon)
  Chronic aspirin ingestion
  Ulcerative colitis
  Oesophageal varices
  Bladder cancer
  Renal cancer
  Chronic urinary tract infection
  Endometrial carcinoma
  Fungating tumours of the skin surface

increased. A bone marrow test shows erythroid hyperplasia and absent or greatly reduced iron stores.

If iron deficiency anaemia is present at the outset in a patient with a solid tumour, it is likely that blood loss is the cause. Possible investigations of the source of blood loss are shown in Table 3.5 but the decision to use any of these tests should be taken in the light of a full history and physical examination.

The treatment of a tumour causing blood loss is, if possible, to eradicate the cancer itself or at least control its growth. Symptomatic treatment with blood transfusion may be necessary. Sometimes, oral iron administration is warranted to replenish iron stores, especially if continued chronic blood loss is likely. Although many and often expensive formulations of iron are available, it is best to use a simple preparation (e.g. ferrous sulphate 200 mg t.d.s).

Infection

This may be an important factor in some tumours, such as lung

85

Table 3.5. Investigations of a patient with iron-deficiency anaemia

Investigations commonly required
  Examination of faeces for occult blood
  Barium meal
  Barium swallow
  Gastroscopy
  Barium enema
  Sigmoidoscopy
  Colonoscopy
  Microscopy of the urine

Investigations less commonly required
  Cystoscopy/pyelography
  Examination of faeces for parasites
  Jejunal biopsy
  Laparotomy for unexplained gastrointestinal trace blood loss

cancer with bronchial obstruction, cancers (bladder and uterus) causing urinary obstruction and ulcerating tumours of the skin, head and neck.

Metastases

Metastatic involvement of the bone marrow occurs in about 20% of all fatal cases of malignant disease. The anaemia is frequently leuco-erythroblastic (characterised by the presence of immature red and white cells in the blood). This type of blood picture in a patient with cancer usually means bone marrow involvement.

Poor nutrition

Disturbance of nutrition caused by anorexia, vomiting, dysphagia and diarrhoea, may contribute to the development of anaemia by impairing intake and reducing absorption of iron and other important haematinics. Although often a contributing factor, this is rarely the sole cause of the anaemia.

Haemolytic anaemia

Acquired haemolytic anaemia is a relatively rare complication of malignancy which is most common in the lymphomas and leukaemia. It does, however, also occur in carcinoma of the stomach, pancreas, prostate and with metastatic carcinoma in bone.

Impaired renal function

This can occur in malignancy but is seldom an important factor.

Anaemia of disseminated malignancy

An anaemia, for which none of the above causes seems to be responsible, develops in some patients. Like the anaemia of chronic infection or renal failure, this results from impaired red blood cell production and increased red blood cell destruction and is, usually, normochromic and normocytic.

Treatment

The treatment of all these types of anaemia is to control or eradicate the underlying tumour. Transfusion of red blood cells should be reserved for patients with symptoms attributable to their anaemia (most patients are not symptomatic unless their haematocrit is less than 25%). Transfusion is not without problems (risk of hepatitis, hypersensitivity, sensitisation and fluid overload) and these should be balanced against the potential benefit. Packed red blood cells are usually preferable to whole blood, in order to reduce the fluid volume infused and the risk of hepatitis. Occasionally, patients sensitised to multiple HLA or white blood cell antigens, may need washed or fresh frozen red blood cells.

Iron and supplemental vitamins are not generally helpful but may be useful in selected instances.

Neutropenia

This is the most common side-effect of cancer chemotherapy and usually develops within 5-10 days of treatment and lasts for about 1 week. It is nearly always reversible but when the neutrophil count falls below $0.5 \times 10^9/l$, the risk of infection is great. Prophylactic antibiotics have not been proven to be of benefit, though clinical trials are continuing. If a patient, after treatment, is likely to become severely neutropenic for more than 3 days, it is wise to keep them in hospital during this time. Some hospitals use sterile environments and regimes to sterilise the skin and gut. Whilst these precautions reduce the infection rate, there is little evidence that they improve the chances of survival and they are often time-consuming and unpleasant for the patient. These types of regimes should, generally, be kept for specific situations, such as bone marrow transplantation, where benefit is demonstrable.

Any patient developing a fever at a time when they may be neutropenic must have an urgent blood count. If this shows a neutrophil count of less than $0.5 \times 10^9/l$ or a total white blood cell count of less than $1.0 \times 10^9/l$, i.v. antibiotics should be started after cultures for infection have been taken (see section 3.2).

Granulocytes for transfusion are now available by centrifugation or filtration but their role in the treatment of neutropenic and bacteraemic patients remains unclear. The commonly used indications for granulocyte transfusion are:

- neutropenia less than $0.2 \times 10^9/l$
- sepsis, especially if there is evidence of worsening infection in spite of appropriate antibiotics
- bone marrow suppression likely to last for more than 5 days

When granulocyte transfusions (more than 10^{10} cells daily) have been used under these conditions in clinical trials, only marginal benefits have been shown and so their routine use cannot be recommended.

Thrombocytopenia

Thrombocytopenia usually occurs together with neutropenia and anaemia and is most commonly the result of cytotoxic drug therapy. Idiopathic thrombocytopenia, hypersplenism and disseminated intravascular coagulation (DIC) are rarer causes during malignancy.

Thrombocytopenia secondary to drug treatment is almost always reversible but there is a risk of haemorrhage during the period of marrow suppression. Spontaneous bleeding commonly only occurs when the platelet count is less than $20 \times 10^9/l$. Aspirin, alcohol and anticoagulants may, however, cause a severe bleed when the platelet count is greater than $20 \times 10^9/l$.

In many patients, the thrombocytopenia is expected and is explained by cytotoxic treatment. Unexpected thrombocytopenia needs investigation which will include:

- bone marrow tests

3.0 General management problems

3.7 Haematological problems

- estimation of spleen size (physical examination, ultrasound or isotope scan)
- tests for DIC, uraemia, liver disease

Patients with severe thrombocytopenia ($< 20 \times 10^9$/l) should be examined daily for fresh purpura and fundal haemorrhages and their urine and stools tested for blood.

Indications for platelet transfusion:

- obvious haemorrhage if platelets $< 20 \times 10^9$/l
- fresh purpura and/or fundal haemorrhages if platelet count is likely to stay low
- pre-surgery
- prophylaxis if there is a high risk of bleeding (e.g. AML induction)
- sudden bleeding or drop in platelets in a patient with a low platelet count (e.g. AML) may be caused by infection

If there is haemorrhage associated with thrombocytopenia, transfusions of platelet concentrates are necessary. Thrombocytopenic patients needing surgery should have pre-operative platelet transfusions to achieve a platelet count of more than 100×10^9/l. If the initial transfusion (usually 6 units) fails to control the haemorrhage, further transfusions should be given until the bleeding stops. In mild cases transfusions, 24 hours apart, will control the problem but a platelet count should be done daily, to see if a rise in platelet count has occurred and to monitor the need for further platelets. If many transfusions are likely to be required over a long period, then HLA-compatible platelets (if available) are preferable.

Immune thrombocytopenia requires treatment of the underlying tumour, steroids and possible splenectomy. Hypersplenism may also require splenectomy.

Thrombosis

Thrombotic phenomena have been recognised as a complication of cancer for many years and were first described by Trousseau. They have been reported in a variety of tumours, as shown in Table 3.6.

Overall, about 1 in 8 patients with cancer have some thrombotic complications. The common problems are recurrent or migratory

3.0 General management problems

3.7 Haematological problems

Table 3.6. Tumours associated with thrombosis

Tumour	Incidence of thrombosis	Proposed mechanism
Pancreas	***	
Stomach	***	
Lung	**	
Breast	*	Chronic DIC
Colon	*	
Ovary	*	
Prostate	*	
Polycythaemia rubra vera	**	
Chronic myelogenous leukaemia	**	Platelet dysfunction + chronic DIC
Thrombocythaemia	*	

thrombophlebitis, arterial embolisation, pulmonary embolism and non-bacterial endocarditis.

The mechanism of thrombosis is not known but numerous coagulation abnormalities have been reported, of which DIC is the most common. In this condition, an exaggerated haemostatic response to tissue injury is initiated, circulating thrombin is generated and fibrin is formed. DIC can comprise 4 phases:

1. As a result of platelet and fibrin deposition in small blood vessels, microthrombi may develop and cause multiple organ failure.
2. Secondary kinin activation and platelet damage occur and can result in metabolic acidosis and hypotension.
3. If severe, there may be marked consumption of platelets and coagulation factors resulting in thrombocytopenia and bleeding.
4. The plasma fibrinolytic system is activated as a secondary response to the activation of the coagulation system and may contribute to the haemorrhagic tendency.

Treatment should be started after consultation with a haematologist and usually comprises:

1. Control of the underlying tumour if possible.

2. Replacement of blood components—fresh whole blood platelets.
3. Interruption of the clotting cycle. This is best achieved by giving heparin 100 units per kg, followed by 10-15 units/kg per hour, by constant i.v. infusion.
4. Frequent checking for a response to therapy as indicated by a rising fibrinogen level and a fall in the fibrin degradation products.

Haemorrhage

Haemorrhage can be caused by multiple factors in patients with cancer. Some of the studies that may be needed to find the cause of an acute bleed are given below.

History

- prior bleeding tendency
- recent drug therapy, especially cytotoxics, anticoagulants and analgesics

Physical examination

- site of bleeding
- purpura, retinal haemorrhages
- signs of liver failure

Laboratory tests

- full blood count
- platelet count
- prothrombin time (PT), partial thromboplastin time (PTT) thrombin time (TT), fibrinogen and fibrinogen degradation product (FDP) tests
- LFTs, U and E
- microbiological studies if indicated

Treatment

The treatment of a haemorrhagic tendency will depend on the cause. Initially, local measures and blood transfusion are required. Specific treatment for the underlying cause is shown in Table 3.7.

Table 3.7. Treatment of various types of haemorrhagic tendency in patients with cancer

Cause	Treatment
Acute promyelocytic leukaemia	Cytotoxic therapy and heparin with blood and platelet transfusion
Waldenstrom's macroglobulinaemia	Plasmapheresis
Marrow replacement causing thrombocytopenia	Cytotoxic therapy
Hypersplenism	Treatment of tumour, splenectomy
Immune thrombocytopenia	Splenectomy, steroids
Cytotoxic chemotherapy	Platelet transfusion
Bleeding gastrointestinal tract tumour	Surgery, radiotherapy
Severe haemoptysis	Radiotherapy
Liver failure	Vitamin K

3.8 Neurological problems

In cancer patients, neurological problems often present difficulties in diagnosis, since there are many possible causes.

1. Many tumours metastasise to the CNS with a variety of clinical presentations.
2. Some tumours (especially bronchial carcinoma) can cause non-metastatic effects on the CNS — the 'paraneoplastic syndromes' (see below).
3. Patients immunosuppressed because of lymphoma or chemotherapy, may develop meningitis with unusual organisms or atypical symptoms (see section 3.2).
4. Tumours may cause metabolic disturbances which in turn may affect the CNS (see section 3.1).
5. Treatment itself may produce neurological symptoms (e.g. vinca alkaloid neuropathy and radiation myelitis).
6. Many cancer patients are elderly and, therefore, at risk from cerebrovascular disease, a risk made worse during episodes of thrombocytopenia.

The problems of differential diagnosis can, therefore, be great and it may be difficult to get a precise answer without complex and sometimes invasive investigation, which may be inappropriate in patients with advanced disease. The more common problems are outlined below but it is worth emphasising 3 conditions that require *urgent* investigation and treatment:

- raised intracranial pressure
- spinal cord compression
- meningitis

Raised intracranial pressure

The classic clinical symptoms of morning headache, nausea and projectile vomiting, may not always be present, particularly if the onset is insidious. Papilloedema is the best confirmatory clinical sign.

In a patient with a known tumour, an intracranial secondary deposit is the most likely cause but other causes include meningitis (infective or malignant) and benign intracranial hypertension. Ideally, the diagnosis should be confirmed by CT scan. If meningism is present a lumbar puncture should only be performed once a space-occupying lesion has been excluded. Treatment is urgent, especially if there are signs of brainstem or cerebellar dysfunction or deteriorating visual acuity. It consists of:

- reducing cerebral oedema: dexamethasone, 4 mg 6-hourly (mannitol i.v., if a very rapid response is needed)
- treating the symptoms: analgesics, anti-emetics
- treating the underlying cause (see below)

Cerebral metastases

These are most common in patients with bronchial, renal and breast carcinoma, malignant melanoma and certain lymphomas. They may present in various ways:

- raised intracranial pressure
- local neurological signs
- fits
- meningitis

The diagnosis should be confirmed by CT or isotope scan or, if there is meningism (and a mass lesion has been excluded), by lumbar puncture.

3.0 General management problems

3.8 Neurological problems

Treatment

1. Dexamethasone, up to 4 mg 6-hourly, will reduce cerebral oedema and the symptoms of raised intracranial pressure and may improve neurological deficit.
2. Whole brain irradiation is the most effective treatment of the tumour but should not be undertaken if the prognosis is poor, because of recurrent primary tumour or other metastases.
3. Systemic chemotherapy is rarely effective, as most drugs do not cross the blood-brain barrier.
4. Intrathecal chemotherapy (see section 4.8) is only effective for meningeal involvement.
5. Surgical excision should only be considered if there is a solitary slow-growing metastasis (e.g. in renal-cell carcinoma) and the tumour elsewhere is treatable or in remission.
6. Anticonvulsants, to prevent fits (see below).

Meningitis

In a cancer patient presenting with signs and symptoms of meningitis, the important differential diagnosis is between infection (bacterial, viral or protozoal), metastasis and haemorrhage (especially if the patient is thrombocytopenic).

Tumour infiltration of the meninges is common in leukaemia and undifferentiated lymphomas but rare in most carcinomas. Clinical features may include:

- signs of raised intracranial pressure
- meningism and photophobia
- pyrexia
- one or more cranial nerve lesions
- extensive radicular disease causing pain or a 'pseudo-Guillain-Barré' syndrome
- transverse myelitis

The diagnosis is made by lumbar puncture: CSF samples should be sent for chemical pathology, bacteriology and virology tests and to an experienced cytologist. The glucose is often reduced, the protein raised and, most important of all, abnormal cells may be demonstrated in a cytocentrifuge preparation. If no abnormal cells are seen but meningeal lymphoma is still suspected, it is worth taking several CSF samples to exclude the diagnosis. These should be examined fresh for lymphocyte surface markers.

3.0 General management problems

3.8 Neurological problems

Treatment of leukaemic or lymphomatous meningitis usually comprises 5 intrathecal injections of methotrexate followed by 5 of cytosine arabinoside given twice weekly and can be monitored by a CSF cell count (see section 4.6). Meningeal carcinomatosis is rarely responsive to cytotoxic therapy but the alkylating agent, thiotepa, can also be given by intrathecal injection. Cranial irradiation can be given concurrently with intrathecal treatment or deferred until evidence of a definite response is seen. Improvement can be dramatic in the lymphomas and leukaemias, provided that there has not been severe neurological damage.

Infective causes of meningitis are treated in the usual manner if of bacterial origin. Tuberculosis should always be remembered as a possible cause. A more serious problem is cryptococcal meningitis, most often seen in children with acute leukaemia. The onset is insidious and the diagnosis often established after several lumbar punctures. The treatment is systemic antifungals, as described in section 3.2. Viral meningitis/encephalitis is also a serious problem, usually associated with disseminated herpes zoster and antiviral agents, such as acyclovir, may be tried, although treatment is often unsuccessful.

Spinal cord compression

This is an emergency, as progression can be rapid. If the diagnosis is suspected, myelography should be undertaken urgently, at which time a sample of CSF can be taken for cytology, biochemistry and bacteriological and glucose analysis.

Extradural deposits are the most common cause, usually from primaries in the breast, lung, prostate or lymphoid tissue. Collapse of vertebral bodies due to metastases, can give a similar picture.

Pain is a common presenting symptom and can be present for months before the first clinical sign. It is frequently useful for local-ising the metastases if the neurological signs are equivocal. If local tenderness is present, an X-ray or bone scan may demonstrate a vertebral deposit.

The advice of a neurosurgeon should be sought urgently. Where a histological diagnosis has not been made and the cord compression is the presenting feature, surgical exploration is essential. If decom-pressive laminectomy is not thought appropriate, local radiotherapy can be given. In addition, dexamethasone, 4 mg 6-hourly, helps to reduce cord oedema. Spastic paraplegia should be avoided at all costs by quick action, as the life expectancy of such patients may often be quite long. Once loss of sphincter control is established, the chances of a good neurological recovery are poor.

Nerve, plexus and root involvement

Direct tumour infiltration of peripheral nerves, plexuses or nerve roots, can occur in many tumours. The initial symptom is normally pain, followed by loss of motor and sensory function. Involvement of nerves and plexuses is usually by direct growth from primary or secondary tumour, and of nerve roots by diffuse meningeal tumour.

Cranial nerves

- head and neck tumours
- orbital tumours
- skull metastases
- lymphomas

Brachial plexus

- supraclavicular or axillary node involvement by carcinoma or lymphoma
- apical lung carcinoma (Pancoast's syndrome)

Sacral plexus

- retroperitoneal tumours
- pelvic tumours (especially of the cervix, or colon carcinomas)

Nerve roots

- multiple: lymphoma, leukaemia
- individual: vertebral bone metastases with pathological fracture (especially myeloma, breast carcinoma)

Peripheral nerves (rare)

- diffuse: lymphoma, leukaemia
- individual: growth from any adjacent metastases

3.0 General management problems

3.8 Neurological problems

Among the more common non-malignant causes of peripheral nerve involvement that should be considered in differential diagnosis are:

- herpes zoster
- drugs (see below)
- Guillain-Barré syndrome
- spondylosis
- prolapsed intervertebral disc
- irradiation (especially brachial plexus)

Treatment

The treatment of choice for malignant involvement is usually local radiotherapy but diffuse involvement by lymphoma or leukaemia will respond to chemotherapy.

Peripheral neuropathy

Peripheral neuropathy should be carefully distinguished by clinical examination from involvement of individual nerves, plexuses or roots, and is rarely caused by direct tumour involvement. In cancer patients, it is most often drug-induced (see section 4.3) but may be caused by a remote effect of the tumour (see paraneoplastic syndromes below).

The most common drugs causing peripheral neuropathy are:

- vinca alkaloids (these may also cause cranial nerve palsies and autonomic neuropathy)
- cisplatin
- procarbazine
- hexamethylmelamine

Drug-induced neuropathy usually recovers slowly once the drug has been discontinued but there may be permanent residual dysfunction.

Myopathy

The most common cause of a true myopathy in cancer patients is prolonged corticosteroid therapy which, typically, causes a proximal myopathy. Myopathy may also be part of a paraneoplastic syndrome (see below).

3.0 General management problems

3.8 Neurological problems

Paraneoplastic syndromes

Some tumours, especially bronchial carcinoma, are associated with non-metastatic neurological dysfunction — the paraneoplastic syndromes. The aetiology of these conditions is obscure. They include:

- peripheral neuropathy — characteristically a segmental demyelination
- myasthenic syndrome (Eaton-Lambert) in which there is no response to anticholinergics but there may be a response to guanidine hydrochloride, 250 mg t.d.s.
- subacute cerebellar degeneration
- transverse myelopathy

Treatment is essentially that of the underlying tumour, following which there is normally improvement.

Fits

These are commonly of the grand mal type but may be Jacksonian in cases of a localised space-occupying lesion. To avoid further brain damage, fits should be controlled with immediate anticonvulsants. Repetitive seizures require:

- diazepam, 5-20 mg i.v. by slow infusion, with careful monitoring of respiratory status
- phenytoin, up to 50 mg/min i.v.
- dexamethasone, 4 mg q.d.s. i.v.

Control is usually maintained with phenytoin, 300 mg daily and serum levels should be monitored.

The following underlying causes should be borne in mind:

- meningeal infection
- intracerebral tumour
- meningeal tumour
- electrolyte disturbances, including low Ca^{2+} or Mg^{2+}
- uraemia
- hypoglycaemia
- liver failure
- anoxia
- intracranial haemorrhage

- intracranial venous thrombosis
- drugs, especially cisplatin

Toxic confusional states

Symptoms may vary from a mild confusional state to deep coma. The following underlying causes should be considered:

- hypercalcaemia (see section 3.1)
- ectopic ADH production (restrict fluids to 1 litre/day and give demeclocycline, 600 mg daily; see section 3.1)
- hyperglycaemia (steroid therapy may worsen diabetes mellitus)
- frontal lobe metastases
- encephalopathy: methotrexate-induced (see section 4.4)
- following cranial irradiation
- drug-related: check sedation, etc.
- infection (see section 3.2)
- hyperviscosity syndrome (myeloma, macroglobulinaemia)

A thorough search should be made for a treatable underlying cause. If a biochemical disorder is found, once the immediate abnormality is improved, the underlying tumour should be treated accordingly. Patients with mild-to-moderate disorientation benefit from familiar surroundings and continuity of care.

3.9 Pain control

Pain is a common, though by no means inevitable, symptom of malignant disease and, therefore, a frequent problem in management.

Causes

The first important step in the management of pain is to make an accurate diagnosis, because the pain may not necessarily be due to the tumour. It may be caused by one or more of the following conditions:

Primary tumours

Direct tumour involvement of the:

- peripheral nerve
- nerve roots or plexus

3.0 General management problems

3.9 Pain control

- spinal cord
- soft tissues
- viscus
- bone

Secondary effect of tumour

- inflammation and oedema
- infection
- obstruction
- pathological fracture
- raised intracranial pressure

Effect of treatment

- post-surgery (especially amputation, mastectomy and thoracotomy)
- chemotherapy-induced phlebitis and tissue damage
- peripheral neuropathy (vinca alkaloids, cisplatin)
- mucositis, oesophagitis (chemotherapy, radiotherapy)
- steroid withdrawal polyarthralgia
- steroid-induced peptic ulcer
- post-irradiation nerve plexus fibrosis and myelopathy

Other important causes

- herpes zoster and post-herpetic neuralgia
- intercurrent illness (e.g. ulcer, angina, prolapsed intervertebral disc)
- intestinal obstruction due to adhesions following laparotomy or radiotherapy

Management

The management of pain depends on the underlying cause.

Surgery

This can be useful in a number of situations:

- pinning pathological fractures of long bones
- bypass or removal of tumour obstruction
- relief of extradural compression of spinal cord or nerve roots

3.0   General management problems

3.9   Pain control

Radiotherapy

This is very useful in controlling pain due to localised tumour infiltration and should always be considered in this situation, unless the prognosis is very poor or the patient is too unwell to tolerate treatment.

Chemotherapy

Chemotherapy can, occasionally, be used to relieve pain directly related to tumour. It is indicated when the tumour has a high chance of being chemosensitive and when radiotherapy is not possible, either because of the number and extent of the sites of disease (e.g. multiple bone metastases) or because of recurrence within an area previously irradiated to tissue tolerance.

Nerve blocks

Nerve blocks are useful where the pain is due to direct infiltration of nerves, plexuses or roots. Of particular use, are brachial plexus, intercostal and coeliac plexus blocks, as well as intrathecal nerve block. The usual procedure involves injection of neurolytic agents such as phenol but analgesia of several weeks duration can result from injection of local anaesthetics. These procedures are specialised and potentially hazardous and are best left to anaesthetists skilled in their use.

Analgesic drugs

These are obviously the mainstay of management of pain but require careful choice and prescribing for maximum benefit and minimum toxicity.

Before prescribing analgesics, it is worth spending time with the patient, not only defining carefully the site, periodicity, quality, duration and severity of pain and recording them for future reference (a body chart may be useful) but, also, assessing the patient's psychological state, social support and awareness of the problem and explaining how the drugs will help.

Many patients worry about becoming addicted to painkillers or that the drugs will become less effective the more they use them and so they will tend to underuse drugs and not take them as instructed. It is important to reassure the patient on these points and to explain that the purpose of the analgesic regime is to keep him as free from pain as possible throughout the day and night, and that there is no virtue in enduring pain.

The most important principle of prescribing analgesics is regular administration to *prevent* pain occurring, rather than giving them only when the pain occurs. A lower dose can often be used to keep a pain at bay than to treat it once it has started. For most drugs, the length of effect is such that regular 4-hourly administration is needed (see below). In addition to their regular dose of analgesics, patients should be prescribed a reserve supply of a stronger analgesic or advised to take a larger dose any time there is a sudden exacerbation of pain.

As far as possible, analgesics should be given orally and parenteral administration reserved for emergency relief of pain or when oral drugs cannot be tolerated, which should be only for a few days at most.

Non-narcotic analgesics should be tried first in patients with mild pain:

- aspirin, 300-1200 mg 4-hourly
- paracetamol, 500-1000 mg 4-hourly

Aspirin may cause dyspepsia and gastrointestinal bleeding and an enteric-coated formulation may be preferable. Very high doses may cause tinnitus and hyperventilation.

Either aspirin, or one of the other potent non-steroidal anti-inflammatory drugs, are particularly useful in the management of *bone metastases.* The ones most commonly used are:

- phenylbutazone, 100 mg 8-hourly
- indomethacin, 25-50 mg 8-hourly (may also be given as suppositories)

There are a variety of different formulations of these drugs and it is best to prescribe only drugs with which one is familiar. If the pain is not well controlled by a non-narcotic drug at adequate dosage, a weak narcotic should be given.

Weak narcotic analgesics should be used for controlling moderate pain and when non-narcotic drugs have failed.

3.0 General management problems

3.9 Pain control

The most useful drugs are:

- codeine, 30-60 mg 4-hourly
- dihydrocodeine, 30-60 mg 4-hourly

Both of these produce, to a lesser extent, the side-effects of strong opiates (see below) but constipation is usually the most troublesome.

Distalgesic (dextroproxyphene 32.5 mg and paracetamol 325 mg) is very popular with patients and doctors but there is little evidence that the dextropropoxyphene contributes to the analgesic effect of the paracetamol at the dose used.

Pethidine and pentazocine are not good analgesics orally and do not have a place in the management of chronic pain. Pethidine also has a short-lived effect given intramuscularly and pentazocine has an unacceptably high incidence of psychological side-effects (especially agitation and hallucinations).

Strong narcotic analgesics are often required when other drugs fail. The most commonly used are morphine and diamorphine and these are best given orally, 3-4 hourly, in a simple solution in chloroform water. Complex formulations including cocaine and chlorpromazine, are unnecessary and have the problem that to increase the dose of analgesic the dose of the other components is increased as well, which may be undesirable.

Cocaine has been shown not to significantly increase the analgesic effect and tolerance to it seems to occur rapidly. It is, therefore, not indicated for routine use with strong narcotics.

Morphine is also available as a 10 mg or 30 mg slow release tablet (MST1 and MST3) which can be given 8- to 12-hourly.

Other strong narcotics include:

- dextromoramide, 5-10 mg: short duration of action (1-2 hours), may be useful for acute exacerbations
- dipipanone, 10-20 mg, 4- to 6-hourly: only available in combination with cyclizine 30 mg (Diconal), so doses cannot be increased beyond 2 tablets
- methadone, 10 mg upwards, 8- to 12-hourly: sedative and tends to accumulate; use with care in elderly
- phenazocine, 5 mg upwards, 4- to 6-hourly: give sublingually — bitter taste

When oral analgesics are not tolerated, the following can be used:

* morphine suppositories, 10-20 mg
* diamorphine injection — parenteral agent of choice, because very soluble and up to 300 mg can be dissolved in 0.5 ml

Consider continuous i.v. or subcutaneous infusion of diamorphine in patients with very severe, poorly controlled pain.

Side-effects of narcotics include:

* sedation: great variability in individual susceptibility; tends to decrease with continued use
* nausea: tends to improve after 7-10 days, some patients may require regular anti-emetics
* constipation: almost inevitable, regular laxatives should be given with all narcotics
* addiction and tolerance: *not* a significant problem in patients with chronic pain
* respiratory depression: use with care in patients with respiratory failure

Phenothiazines (e.g. promazine and chlorpromazine) may be used in some patients to potentiate the analgesic effect, suppress nausea and vomiting or increase sedation.

The approximate dose equivalence of narcotic analgesics is shown in Table 3.8.

3.10   Pregnancy and contraception

Pregnancy in a woman requiring treatment for malignant disease presents obvious problems. The management has to be individualised and requires much careful thought and discussion. In general, if systemic chemotherapy or abdominal radiotherapy is planned, therapeutic abortion should be advised for pregnancies in the first trimester and, in the third trimester it may, sometimes, be possible to delay treatment until after delivery. In the middle trimester, therapeutic abortion is usually the most appropriate course, although in exceptional circumstances, such as Hodgkin's disease confined to areas above the diaphragm, definitive radiotherapy can be given with minimal risk to the fetus.

Table 3.8. Dose equivalence of narcotic analgesics (after Twycross, 1978)

Drug

Diamorphine hydrochloride (orally)	10 mg
Diamorphine hydrochloride (i.m.)	5 mg
Morphine sulphate (orally)	15 mg
Dipipanone	30 mg
Methadone	10 mg (long half-life, accumulates)
Dextromoramide	5 mg (short-lived effect)
Phenazocine	3 mg

All anticancer drugs are potentially teratogenic and so women receiving them should take contraceptive measures. Patients treated with alkylating agents may be rendered temporarily or permanently infertile (see section 4.4) but, if normal menstrual function returns after chemotherapy, normal pregnancy can still take place and the risks of malformation seem to be small. Patients often seek advice on starting a family after a course of chemo-therapy. A minimum period of 1 year after cytotoxic drug adminis-tration is a good general guide but the advice given should also be tempered by the likelihood of recurrence of the particular tumour.

Men receiving chemotherapy should also take contraceptive precautions because of the teratogenic risks, although many will be rendered azoospermic (see section 4.3).

3.11 Psychological problems

Psychological disturbance is very frequent in patients with malignant disease. Anxiety and/or depression often occur as a reaction to the illness or treatment but may require little or no specific therapy, apart from a sympathetic ear and plenty of time to discuss problems and answer questions.

Anger and denial are psychological defences commonly employed in coping with the stress of illness and it is important to recognise them as such when they occur in patients or relatives.

Major psychotic episodes are uncommon but may occur in a pre-morbid personality. A number of patients are unable to cope for a

number of reasons and become very anxious or depressed.
Sympathy and reassurance are not sufficient for such patients, who
may well benefit from anxiolytic or antidepressant drugs or a
psychiatric referral.

There are a number of causes of an organic brain syndrome that
may vary from a mild confusional state to coma or may, occasionally, manifest itself as depression or major psychosis. The following
should be considered and excluded by investigation, where
appropriate:

- anoxia
- pyrexia
- anaemia
- hypercalcaemia
- uraemia
- liver failure
- inappropriate ADH secretion
- drugs, especially opiates, procarbazine, asparaginase, steroids
- brain metastases (especially frontal lobe)
- non-metastatic organic brain syndromes (e.g. lymphoma-
  associated subacute sclerosing panencephalitis)

A common problem is that of whether patients should or should not
be told the diagnosis. It is impossible and inappropriate to be
dogmatic about this but, probably, a very high proportion of
patients know or strongly suspect that they have cancer, even
though they have never been directly told and, in general, an
atmosphere of frankness and open discussion helps everyone
involved. It is, however, as wrong to force information on a patient
who does not want to know, as it is to withhold it from a patient
who does. Equally, it places an intolerable strain on one member of
a close family unit to have to withhold information from the others.

3.12   Fungating tumours and fistulae

These are common problems in advanced malignant disease,
especially with tumours of the head and neck, breast and female
genital tract.

Surgery is the definitive treatment of first choice but is often not
possible for technical reasons when tumours are advanced. Radiotherapy may be used in addition or when surgery is impossible and

chemotherapy tried only when other modalities have failed and when there is a reasonable chance of response.

Offensive smell is a common symptomatic problem. This can be helped by regular cleaning and dressing, using a standard antiseptic such as chlorhexidine or povidone-iodine. A short course of broad spectrum antibiotics may be useful if there is deep infection in any area that cannot be cleaned, and metronidazole is indicated, particularly if there is a large bowel fistula with a risk of anaerobic infection. Dressing pads containing activated charcoal are available, if smell is a persistent problem.

Vaginal discharge associated with fistula may be helped by metronidazole orally or hydrargaphen pessaries, in addition to regular local cleansing.

The normal skin around external fistulae should be protected with a suitable barrier and excess discharge managed, either with regularly changed absorbent dressings or, where feasible, a stoma bag.

3.13 Alopecia

The majority of cytotoxic drugs cause some degree of hair loss, in particular the anthracyclines and alkylating agents given intravenously in high doses (see section 4.3). Alopecia is, therefore, a common problem and one that is often disproportionally worrying to the patient.

The first thing to do is to reassure the patient that the hair usually comes out gradually over a few weeks after starting chemotherapy, rather than suddenly and that it will start to grow again, as soon as treatment is stopped (and sometimes even while treatment continues). The regrown hair is sometimes different in texture and colour from the original hair.

Wigs are available on prescription for patients receiving chemotherapy or cranial irradiation and arrangements should be made for ordering and fitting at the beginning of any treatment likely to cause alopecia, before hair loss has started, so that colour and styles can be matched, and also so that the patient has the wig available as soon as hair loss starts. On the whole, wigs for women are more cosmetically acceptable than those for men.

3.13   Alopecia

Attempts have been made to prevent alopecia by applying a scalp
tourniquet or by cooling of the scalp for a period of time during and
after the injection, to prevent the drug reaching the hair follicles.
Special helmets to keep ice-packs or equivalent 'cool-bags' in place
have been devised. These techniques can be effective, if the drug
has a short peak blood level but are cumbersome, uncomfortable
and time-consuming (the ischaemia must be maintained for up to
1 hour) and, therefore, not suited to routine use in a busy chemotherapy clinic. There is also the theoretical risk that tumour cells in
the scalp area are not being treated adequately, which may lead to
subsequent relapse.

3.0 General management problems

Notes

3.0 General management problems

Notes
_____

4.0 Cytotoxic drugs

4.0 Cytotoxic drugs

4.1 Index of cytotoxic drugs and hormonal agents

Cytotoxic drugs generally have a low therapeutic ratio, so a thorough understanding of their safe administration and their potential toxicities is essential to good patient management. It is not within the scope of this book to recommend specific drugs or combinations for all tumours, as chemotherapy is often a controversial and, sometimes, experimental area. In Appendix I we have, however, listed a number of commonly used combinations, with appropriate references.

In the first three sections of this chapter the cytotoxic drugs are listed and described. First, in section 4.1, there is a list of cytotoxic drugs and hormonal agents, arranged in alphabetical order, including alternative and proprietary names, with a reference to the page on which further information is given. A number of investigational agents are included in this list for the sake of completeness, but further information is not given.

Section 4.2 lists the drugs in alphabetical order of approved or most commonly used names. For each drug, information is given on the group to which the drug belongs, dosage, mode of administration, precautions, toxicity, storage, interactions and, where known, on its metabolism. *The information on dosage is necessarily only an approximate guide*, not precise prescribing information, as doses will vary with different combinations. Reference should always be made to the regime employed.

In particular, *the upper dose levels of many drugs can be associated with severe toxicity* and should only be administered under the supervision of those experienced in their use.

A number of drugs which are not yet approved for use and, therefore, not freely available in the UK, are listed and are marked with an asterisk.

Section 4.3 is a table of toxicities, which lists the most commonly encountered toxicities under body systems and the drugs causing them, with an approximate rating of frequency. Very rare toxicities or those reported but with a dubious relationship to the drug, are not included.

4.0 Cytotoxic drugs

4.1 Index of cytotoxic and hormonal agents

4.0 Cytotoxic drugs

4.1 Index of cytotoxic and hormonal agents

4.0 Cytotoxic drugs

4.1 Index of cytotoxic and hormonal agents

4.0 Cytotoxic drugs

4.1/4.2   Index/List of cytotoxic and hormonal agents

4.2   Alphabetical list of cytotoxic and hormonal agents

     *   Investigational agent not freely available in the UK

Toxicity rating scale:

+ + + +	inevitable	+ +	infrequent
+ + +	common	+	rare

Doses are an approximate guide, *not* precise prescribing information. Always consult the dosage recommended in the particular regime.

actinomycin D
(Dactinomycin, Cosmegen, Lyovac)
Group: Antibiotic

Dosage		0.015 mg/kg per day for 3-6 days. Usual max. daily dose 0.6 mg/m²
Administration		i.v. bolus into fast-running N. saline infusion
Precautions		Avoid extravasation
Toxicity	+ + + +	Tissue necrosis
		Phlebitis

Toxicity *cont.*	+ + +	Nausea and vomiting
		Myelosuppression (nadir at 10-14 days; recovery 16-20 days)
		Mucositis
	+	Alopecia
		Radiation recall
Monitoring tests		Full blood count and liver function tests
Metabolism and excretion		50-90% excreted in the bile, 10-20% in the urine (consider dose reduction for liver functional impairment)
Storage		Powder—500 μg vials, refrigerated, away from light
		Solution—refrigerated, 24 hours
Interactions		Adriamycin, mithramycin

Adriamycin
(doxorubicin, 14-hydroxydaunomycin)
Group: Antibiotic

Dosage		1-2 mg/kg or 40-70 mg/m², usually given as a single intravenous injection once every 3 weeks. Total dose should not exceed 450 mg/m²
Administration		i.v. bolus into fast running N. saline infusion
Precautions		Avoid extravasation
		Avoid skin contact (wear gloves and goggles when preparing and injecting)
		Dose reduction if abnormal liver function (see below)
Toxicity	+ + + +	Tissue necrosis
		Phlebitis
		Complete alopecia
	+ + +	Nausea and vomiting
		Myelosuppression (nadir at 9-14 days; recovery 16-20 days)
		Mucositis
		Pigmentation
		Urine appears red for up to 24 hours after injection

4.0 Cytotoxic drugs

4.2 Alphabetical list of cytotoxic and hormonal agents

Toxicity *cont.*	+ +	Nail changes
		Pyrexia/rigors
	+	Cardiomyopathy—increasing incidence at total doses of greater than 450 mg/m²
		Ocular
		Radiation recall
		Encephalopathy
Monitoring tests		Full blood count and liver function tests. Check cumulative dose does not exceed 450 mg/m²
Metabolism and excretion		Enterohepatic: consider dose reduction or omission if liver function tests abnormal (Bilirubin 20-50 μmol/l 50% reduction, >50 μmol/l 75% reduction)
Storage		Powder—10 mg, 50 mg vials, refrigerated
		Solution—refrigerated, away from light, 48 hours
Interactions		Actinomycin, azathioprine, 6-mercaptopurine, mithramycin, barbiturates, hypoglycaemic agents

aminoglutethimide
(Orimeten)
Group: Hormonal agent: anti-adrenal

Dosage		250 mg, t.d.s. or q.d.s. continuously, together with dexamethasone, 2 mg t.d.s. or hydrocortisone, 20 mg b.d.
Administration		Orally, 250 mg tablets
Precautions		Simultaneous glucocorticoid administration essential
		Discontinue in the event of inter-current infection, trauma, etc.
		Increase dose slowly over 3-4 weeks when starting treatment, especially in elderly
Toxicity	+ + +	Sedation (can be severe, especially in elderly—introduce drug slowly)

Toxicity *cont.*	Rash (mild, usually transient, even if drug continued)
	Adrenal insufficiency (ensure adequate glucocorticoid replacement—add fludrocortisone, 0.1 mg alternate days, if necessary)
Monitoring test	Urea and electrolytes, BP lying and standing
Storage	Room temperature

androgens
Group: Hormonal agents

Drugs, dosage and administration	testosterone (Sustanon '250', 30 mg, 100 mg amp.), 30-100 mg, every 4 weeks, i.m.
	nandrolone phenylpropionate (Durabolin, 25 mg amp., 25 mg, 50 mg syringes), 25-50 mg/week, i.m.
	nandrolone decanoate (Deca-Durabolin 25 mg, 50 mg syringes, 25 mg, 50 mg, 100 mg amps), 25-50 mg every 3 weeks, i.m.
	oxymethalone (Anapolon, 50 mg tabs), 50-100 mg/day, orally
	orostanolone (Masteril, 100 mg amp.) 300 mg/week, i.m.
	fluoxymestrone (Ultrandren, 5 mg tabs), 30 mg/day, orally
Precautions	Ensure i.m. injections not given i.v. or s.c.
	Contraindicated in severe renal failure or heart failure
Toxicity + + + +	Virilisation
+ + +	Nausea and vomiting
+ +	Oedema (mild)
	Intrahepatic cholestatic jaundice, (testosterone and methyl derivatives only)
Storage	See manufacturers' literature for individual drugs

4.0 Cytotoxic drugs

4.2 Alphabetical list of cytotoxic and hormonal agents

asparaginase*
(Colaspase, Crasnitin)
Group: Enzyme

Dosage		Variable, e.g. 20 000 i.v./m² weekly or 4000 i.v./m², daily × 14
Administration		i.v. infusion over >30 min in N. saline
Precautions		i.m. injection in <2 ml N. saline
		To prevent acute anaphylactic reactions, skin test with 0.1 ml solution (20 i.u.) before each course
		Observe for at least 1 hour after
Toxicity	+ + +	injection
		Pyrexia and rigors
		Hypersensitivity (usually mild and controlled by antihistamines)
		Hepatic (usually transient elevation of enzymes)
		Encephalopathy (occasionally coma)
	+ +	Hyperglycaemia
		Nausea and vomiting
	+	Renal dysfunction
		Myelosuppression
Monitoring tests		Full blood count, liver function tests
Storage		Dry—refrigerated, 4 years; room temperature, 2 years
		Solution—refrigerated, 3 weeks
Interactions		Vincristine, hypoglycaemic agents

5-azacytidine*
(NSC-102, 816)
Group: Anti-metabolite

Dosage	100-200 mg/m² biweekly i.v.
	150-400 mg/m² × 5 i.v., every 21 days or, preferably, as a continuous infusion
	250-500 mg/m² i.v.
Administration	i.v. bolus + N. saline flush
	Continuous i.v. infusion in lactated Ringer's solution
	Subcutaneously

Toxicity	+ + +	Myelosuppression
		Nausea and vomiting (less with infusions)
		Diarrhoea
	+ +	Hepatotoxicity (coma +): consider omitting or reducing dose if severe impairment of liver function
	+	Neuromuscular
		Fever
		Hypotension
		Skin rash
		Rhabdomyolysis
		Hypophosphataemia

Monitoring tests — Full blood count and liver function tests

Storage — Undiluted drug is stable for 2 years if refrigerated. Supplied in 100 mg vials. Reconstitute with 19.9 ml of saline for injection (*do not* use 5% dextrose in water). Stable for 30 mins. If an infusion is to be used, reconstitute in lactated Ringer's solution where it is stable for 4 hours

Interactions — Pyrazofurin

bleomycin
(Blenoxane)
Group: Antibiotic

Dosage — 15 mg/m², i.m., once a week or 15-30 mg/m², i.v. infusion daily, for 5 days or 1 mg/day, continuous s.c.
Total dosage should not exceed 500 mg but caution should be exercised at total dosages greater than 250 mg

Administration — i.v. bolus in 5-10 ml water or N. saline
i.m. } dissolved in 0.5-1 ml of
s.c. } 1% lignocaine
intracavitary (see section 4.15)

Precautions — Check total dose is less than 500 mg

Precautions *cont.*		Avoid high concentration oxygen administration
Toxicity	+ + + +	Erythema and pigmentation of skin
	+ + +	Pyrexia/rigors (starts 3-6 hours; may be prevented with anti-histamines or corticosteroids)
		Hyperkeratosis
		Pneumonitis and pulmonary fibrosis (dose-limiting, exacerbated by oxygen administration)
		Nail changes
		Alopecia
		Mucositis
	+ +	Radiation recall
	+	Nausea and vomiting
		Phlebitis
Monitoring tests		Clinical examination of the respiratory system and chest X-ray. If lung function tests are used, carbon monoxide transfer is the most sensitive indicator of pulmonary toxicity
Metabolism and excretion		Renal excretion
Storage		Powder—3 mg, 15 mg amp., room temperature
		Solution—stable 24 hours at room temperature

busulphan
(Myleran)
Group: Alkylating agent

Dosage		Continuously, 0.5-10 mg daily, according to FBC
		Intermittently, 50-250 mg, as a single dose
Precautions		May cause prolonged myelo-suppression
Administration		Orally, 0.5 mg, 2 mg tablets
Toxicity	+ + + +	Myelosuppression (nadir 2-4 weeks; recovery 4-8 weeks)
	+ + +	Infertility and amenorrhoea
		Pigmentation
	+	Gynaecomastia

Toxicity *cont.*	Cataracts
	Nausea and vomiting
	Pulmonary fibrosis
Monitoring tests	Regular full blood count
Metabolism and excretion	Excreted in the urine as methane-sulfonic acid
Storage	Room temperature

carmustine
(BCNU, BiCNU)
Group: Nitrosourea

Dosage		Up to 200 mg/m² i.v., every 6-8 weeks
Administration		i.v. infusion over 15-45 min in 100-250 ml 5% dextrose
		Flush with N. saline
Precautions		Follow carefully the manufacturer's instructions for making solutions. Dissolve the powder in each vial in 3 ml of absolute alcohol followed by 27 ml sterile water. Discard any vials with oily deposit indicating overheating and decomposition
Toxicity	+ + + +	Tissue necrosis
		Nausea and vomiting (severe—lasts 6-8 hours)
		Phlebitis (pain at injection site and up the vein—try infusion 5 ml 0.5% lignocaine)
	+ + +	Myelosuppression (moderate to severe: nadir at 3-4 weeks; recovery by 5-7 weeks)
	+ +	Facial flushing (lasts up to 2 hours)
		Hepatic (transient elevation of enzymes)
Monitoring tests		Full blood count
Storage		Dry—refrigerated, up to 2 years; never store at >27°C
		Solution—use as soon as possible, do not store
Metabolism and excretion		Rapid biotransformation—slow urinary excretion of metabolites
		Crosses to CSF
Interactions		Cimetidine

4.0 Cytotoxic drugs

4.2 Alphabetical list of cytotoxic and hormonal agents

chlorambucil
(Leukeran)
Group: Alkylating agent

Dosage		5-15 mg, daily continuous treatment or, occasionally, 20-100 mg/day, intermittently
Administration		Orally, 2 mg, 5 mg tablets
Toxicity	+ + +	Myelosuppression
	+	Nausea and vomiting
		Indigestion
		Hepatic
		Pulmonary
Metabolism and excretion		Unknown, probably extensive metabolism and renal excretion of metabolites
Storage		Room temperature

chlorozotocin*
Group: Nitrosourea

Dosage		120 mg/m^2 i.v., every 6 weeks
Administration		i.v. bolus + flush with N. saline
Precautions		Avoid extravasation
Toxicity	+ + + +	Myelosuppression (nadir at 4 weeks recovery by 6-8 weeks)
		Nausea and vomiting (mild 2-6 hours)
Monitoring tests		Full blood count
Metabolism and excretion		50-60% excretion in the urine as metabolites
Storage		Dry—refrigerated, 18 months Solution—refrigerated, 24 hours

cisplatin
(Cisplatinum, Cis DDP, Neoplatin)
Group: Miscellaneous

Dosage	50-120 mg/m^2 i.v., every 3-4 weeks, or 15-20 mg/m^2, daily × 5
Administration	i.v. infusion in 1-2 l N. saline or 5% dextrose, at a rate of 1 mg/min (see p. 176)
Precautions	Check renal function (serum creatinine, or creatinine

Precautions *cont.*		clearance) before each course
		Establish diuresis of > 150 ml/hour before administration, and maintain for 6 hours after — keep up i.v. fluids until oral fluids tolerated (see section 4.11)
		Use mannitol (*not* loop diuretics), to enhance diuresis
Toxicity	+ + + +	Nausea and vomiting (severe lasts 12-24 hours)
	+ + +	Ototoxicity
		Myelosuppression (nadir at 3 weeks; recovery by 4 weeks)
		Renal failure (check renal function; ensure diuresis)
		Diarrhoea
		Hypomagnesaemia (very common biochemically, rarely symptomatic)
	+ +	Hypocalcaemia (rarely symptomatic)
		Neuropathy
		Fits
	+	Papillitis
Monitoring tests		Full blood count, urea and electrolytes, creatinine clearance, audiometry
Metabolism and excretion		Excretion mainly renal (reduce dose or omit if renal function impaired)
Storage		Dry — refrigerated, away from light, 2 years
		Solution — room temperature, 24 hours
Interactions		Cephalothin, loop diuretics, gentamicin

cyclophosphamide

(Endoxana, Cytoxan)
Group: Alkylating agent

Dosage	50-200 mg orally, daily, or 300-600 mg/m² i.v., every 3 weeks
Administration	i.v. bolus + N. saline flush

Administration *cont.*		Orally, 50 mg tablets
Precautions		Patients should increase fluid intake (>3 l/day) to avoid cystitis
Toxicity	+ + +	Myelosuppression (nadir 1-2 weeks; recovery by 3-5 weeks)
		Alopecia
		Sterility
		Nausea and vomiting (especially with high doses i.v.)
		Haemorrhagic cystitis (consider mesnum; see section 4.12)
	+ +	Mucositis
		Amenorrhoea
		Cardiomyopathy (only with high-dose therapy)
	+	SIADH
		Pulmonary fibrosis
Monitoring tests		Full blood count
Metabolism and excretion		Renal excretion. Activated in liver
Storage		Tablets—room temperature
		Powder—100 mg, 200 mg, 500 mg, 1000 mg vials, room temperature
		Solution—refrigerated, 24 hours
Interactions		Allopurinol; anaesthetic agents; barbiturates; chloramphenicol; chloroquine, corticosteroids; dapsone, hypoglycaemic drugs; N-M blockers

cytosine arabinoside
(Cytosar, Ara C, cytarabine)
Group: Antimetabolite

Dosage	30-200 mg/m² i.v. or i.m. or s.c., daily for 1-7 days, every 2-4 weeks
	50 mg/m² intrathecally, once or twice a week
Administration	i.v. bolus + N. saline flush
	i.m.
	s.c., in 0.5 ml of diluent
	Intrathecal (see section 4.14)

Precautions		Reduce dose if severe liver dysfunction
Toxicity	+ + +	Myelosuppression (nadir at 5-12 days; recovery at 14-16 days)
	+ +	Nausea and vomiting
		Mucositis
		Diarrhoea
	+	Facial flushing
		Abdominal pain
Monitoring tests		Full blood count
Metabolism and excretion		Metabolised in the liver to uracil arabinoside; 90% excreted in the urine as this inactive metabolite
Storage		Powder — 100 mg vials, refrigerated
		Solution — refrigerated, 48 hours

dacarbazine

(DTIC, imidazole carboxamide)
Group: Miscellaneous; alkylating agent (?)

Dosage		2-4.5 mg/kg daily × 10 } every 3-4 weeks
		or 250 mg/m² daily × 5 }
		or 850 mg/m² }
Administration		i.v. bolus in 10 ml N. saline over 1 min, with N. saline flush
		i.v. infusion in 100-200 ml 5% dextrose or N. saline over 15-30 min, with flush
Precautions		Avoid exposure to light
		Avoid extravasation
Toxicity	+ + + +	Myelosuppression (nadir at 3-4 weeks)
		Nausea and vomiting (severe, 1-12 hours)
	+ + +	Phlebitis
	+ +	Pyrexia/rigors (especially after large single dose, starts *c.* day 7, lasts 7-21 days)
		Tissue necrosis
Monitoring tests		Full blood count
Metabolism and excretion		Mainly hepatic
Storage		Dry — refrigerated, away from light, 4 months

| Storage *cont.* | Solution — 200-500 ml N. saline or 5% dextrose, avoid exposure to light, use as soon as possible |

daunorubicin
(Rubidomycin, Daunomycin, Cerubidin)
Group: Antibiotic

Dosage	1-3 mg/kg or 50-100 mg/m², given as a single injection once every 3 weeks. Total dose should not exceed 600 mg/m²
Administration	i.v. bolus into fast-running N. saline infusion
Precautions	Avoid extravasation
	Avoid skin contact (wear gloves and goggles when preparing and injecting)
	Reduce dose if abnormal liver function (see below)
Toxicity + + + +	Alopecia
	Tissue necrosis
+ + +	Phlebitis
	Nausea and vomiting
	Myelosuppression (nadir at 9-14 days; recovery 16-21 days)
	Red urine for up to 24 hours after administration
	Mucositis
+ +	Cardiomyopathy — increasing risk after total dose of 600 mg/m²
Monitoring tests	Full blood count and liver function tests. Check total dose
Metabolism and excretion	Enterohepatic. If bilirubin level 20-50 μmol/l, 50% dose reduction; if <50 μmol/l, 75% dose reduction
Storage and dilution	Powder — 20 mg vials, refrigerated, away from light
	Solution — refrigerate, 24 hours
Interactions	Azathioprine, 6-mercaptopurine, mithramycin, barbiturates

4.2 Alphabetical list of cytotoxic and hormonal agents

---

etoposide
(VP16-213, Vepesid)
Group: Epipodophyllotoxin

Dosage	i.v. 200 mg/m² weekly, or 60-100 mg/m² daily × 5, every 3-4 weeks
	Orally, twice i.v. dosage
Administration	i.v. infusion in 250-500 ml N. saline (*not* 5% dextrose) over 30-45 min
	Orally, 100 mg capsules
Precautions	Avoid extravasation
	Avoid rapid infusion
	Do not dilute in 5% dextrose
Toxicity +++	Myelosuppression (nadir at 2 weeks; recovery by 3 weeks)
++	Alopecia
	Nausea and vomiting (with oral capsules +++)
	Hypotension (occurs only with rapid infusion)
Monitoring tests	Full blood count
Metabolism and excretion	Mainly excreted in urine, partly in bile
Storage	Intact vials—room temperature, avoid light, 3 years
	Capsules—room temperature, 2 years

5-fluorouracil
(5-FU)
Group: Antimetabolite

Dosage	500-1000 mg/m² i.v. or orally, weekly
Administration	i.v. bolus + N. saline flush
	Topical use as an ointment (see section 4.16)

Toxicity	+ + +	Myelosuppression
		Pigmentation
	+ +	Nausea and vomiting
		Phlebitis
		Mucositis
		Diarrhoea
	+	Alopecia
		Skin rash
		Cerebellar ataxia
		Malabsorption
		Ocular
Monitoring tests		Full blood count
Metabolism and excretion		Entero-hepatic circulation. Only 15% excreted by the kidney
Storage		Stable at room temperature, may precipitate if refrigerated. Supplied in 250 mg vials (5 ml) and as an ointment
Interactions		Methotrexate

folinic acid
(Leucovorin, citrovorum factor)

Dosage	30 mg 6-hourly for 12-48 hours, starting 24 hours after methotrexate
Administration	Orally, 15 mg tablets
	i.m.
	i.v. bolus injection
Indications	Used to 'rescue' bone marrow and mucosal surfaces from toxicity of methotrexate, especially after high-dose treatment or in the presence of renal failure. Ideally, monitor serum methotrexate levels and give folinic acid if levels greater than 10^{-3}M at 24 hours, 10^{-6}M at 48 hours and 10^{-7}M at 72 hours (see section 4.10)

4.2 Alphabetical list of cytotoxic and hormonal agents

hexamethylmelamine
(NSC-13875, HMM)
Group: Possible alkylating agent (though active in alkylating agent failures), possible antimetabolite.

Dosage		Orally 300 mg/m² per day (or 8 mg/kg day) Can be used indefinitely if tolerated. An intermittent 21 days on and 21 days off regime is often more acceptable to patients. Capsules of 50 mg and 100 mg
Toxicity	+ + +	nausea and vomiting (often dose-limiting)
	+ +	myelosuppression
	+	neurotoxicity (may be dose-limiting): paraesthesia: sleep disturbance, hallucinations depression, Parkinson-like syndrome, with ataxia. Some investigators report that pyridoxine (100 mg t.d.s.) with a lower dose of HMM may allow continued use of the drug
Monitoring tests		Full blood count
Metabolism and excretion		Rapidly N-methylated in the liver. Metabolites excreted in urine
Storage		Store in tightly sealed bottle (containing desiccant) at room temperature (22°C). Stable for at least two years

hydroxyurea
(Hydrea)
Group: Miscellaneous

Dosage	20-30 mg/kg, continuously, according to blood count or 80 mg/kg every third day
Administration	Orally, 500 mg capsules
Precautions	Hygroscopic, keep bottles tightly closed

Toxicity	+ + +	Myelosuppression (nadir at 10 days)
		Nausea and vomiting (usually mild)
	+	Mucositis
		Pigmentation
		Nail changes
Monitoring tests		Full blood count
Metabolism and excretion		Mainly renal
Storage		Room temperature; tightly closed bottles with desiccant
Interactions		Alcohol, anti-emetics, barbiturates, CNS depressants, narcotic analgesics

ifosfamide
(Holoxan, isophosphamide, Mitoxana)
Group: Alkylating agent

Dosage		1000-5000 mg/m² i.v., every 3 weeks
		500-1000 mg/m² per day × 5, every 3 weeks
Administration		i.v. infusion
		i.v. bolus in at least 75 ml water or N. saline + N. saline flush
Precautions		Ensure adequate hydration during and after therapy to maintain high urine output and minimise urothelial toxicity. Ideally, maintain i.v. infusion for 24-48 hours
		Use mesnum (see section 4.12) with high doses or if previous cystitis
Toxicity	+ + + +	Haemorrhagic cystitis. Use mesnum (see section 4.12) and increase fluid intake
	+ + +	Nausea and vomiting
		Alopecia
	+ +	Myelosuppression
		Phlebitis
	+	Sedation
		Nephrotoxicity

Monitoring tests	Full blood count
Metabolism and excretion	Activated by liver microsomal enzymes. Metabolites excreted in urine
Storage	Available in 1 and 3 g vials. Stable, when refrigerated, for 5 years. Diluted in at least 30 ml of water for injection. Stable, when diluted for 1 week at room temperature and 6 weeks under refrigeration. If diluted in common infusion vehicles stable for 7 days at room temperature but use within 8 hours because no bacteriostatic properties
Interaction	Possibly potentiated by phenobarbitone, phenytoin and chloralhydrate

lomustine
(CCNU, CeeNU)
Group: Nitrosourea

Dosage		100-130 mg/m² every 6 weeks
Administration		Orally, 100 mg, 40 mg, 10 mg capsules
Precautions		Avoid giving more often than 6-weekly because of prolonged myelosuppression
Toxicity	+ + +	Myelosuppression (moderate-to-severe: nadir at 3-5 weeks; recovery by 6-10 weeks)
		Nausea and vomiting (can be severe, lasts 2-6 hours)
	+ +	Alopecia
		Mucositis
	+	Pulmonary fibrosis
Monitoring tests		Full blood count
Metabolism and excretion		Liver metabolism and renal clearance. Fat soluble, crosses to CSF
Storage		Room temperature, 2 years

4.0 Cytotoxic drugs

4.2 Alphabetical list of cytotoxic and hormonal agents

melphalan
(Alkeran, L-phenylalanine mustard, L-PAM)
Group: Alkylating agent

Dosage		5 mg/m² orally, daily × 5, every 6 weeks
		15-40 mg/m² orally or i.v. every 6 weeks
Administration		Orally, 2 mg, 5 mg tablets
		i.v. bolus + N. saline flush
Precautions		Orally — ensure given with food
		i.v. — dilute each 100 mg vial with 1 ml of propranolol diluent (supplied) and then 9 ml of water for injection
Toxicity	+ + +	Myelosuppression (nadir at 21-28 days)
	+ +	Nausea and vomiting
		Amenorrhoea
		Sterility
	+	Cystitis
		Mucositis
Monitoring tests		Full blood count
Metabolism and excretion		Mainly excreted in the urine as metabolites (consider dose reduction if renal impairment)
Storage		Available as 2 mg tablets or 100 mg vial for injection with diluent. Stable for 24 hours after reconstitution. Tablets and injection stored away from direct sunlight at room temperature

6-mercaptopurine
(6-MP, Purinethol)
Group: Antimetabolite

Dosage	50-75 mg/m² daily continuous treatment
Administration	Orally, 2 mg tablet
Precautions	Allopurinol blocks metabolism. Reduce dose by at least 50% if given concurrently with allopurinol

4.2 Alphabetical list of cytotoxic and hormonal agents

Toxicity	+ + +	Myelosuppression
	+ +	Nausea and vomiting
		Liver dysfunction
		Mucositis
	+	Skin rash
		Alopecia
Monitoring tests		Full blood count, liver function tests, check if patient is taking allopurinol
Metabolism and excretion		Oxidation in liver to inactive form; 50% excreted in the urine in 24 hours (consider dose reduction for renal impairment)
Storage		Tablets stable at room temperature
Interactions		Allopurinol

methotrexate
(Amethopterin)
Group: Antimetabolite

Dosage	Orally, continuous 2.5-10 mg/m² per day
	Intermittently, 25-50 mg/m², twice weekly
	i.v. 25-50 mg/m², twice weekly
	High-dose i.v. with folinic acid rescue >200 mg/m² every 1-3 weeks (see section 4.10 for details)
	Intrathecal, 5.0-12.5 mg once or twice weekly
Precautions	Modify dose if renal impairment
	Folinic acid rescue must be given if dose >200 mg/m² (see folinic acid, p. 172)
	May accumulate in effusions and cause prolonged toxicity. Drainage essential before giving high dose
Administration	Orally, 2.5 mg, 10 mg tablets
	i.v. bolus + N. saline flush or infusion
	Intrathecal (see section 4.14)
	Intracavitary (see section 4.15)

Toxicity	+ + +	Myelosuppression (nadir at 7-10 days; recovery at 14-16 days)
		Mucositis
		Nausea and vomiting (high dose)
	+ +	Diarrhoea
		Skin rash
		Cerebral atrophy (see section 4.4)
		Renal dysfunction (high dose)
	+	Alopecia
		Pneumonitis
		Malabsorption
		Ocular
		Liver dysfunction
		Osteoporosis

Monitoring tests — Full blood count, liver function tests, renal function; methotrexate levels if using high dose

Metabolism and excretion — 75% excreted unchanged in urine in first 5 hours. Consider dose reduction if renal impairment and only use high dose if renal function normal

Storage — Tablets—room temperature
Powder—500 mg vials, room temperature
Solution—5 mg, 50 mg vials, room temperature
Opened vials and reconstituted solution—refrigerated, 24 hours

Interactions — 5-fluorouracil, alcohol, aspirin, cephalothin, corticosteroids, hypoglycaemic agents, probenecid, sulphonamides

mithramycin
(Mithracin)
Group: Antibiotic

Dosage — 1.0-1.5 mg/m² per day, for 5-10 days
Hypercalcaemia: 25 μg/kg, daily, for 3-4 days, every 10-14 days

Administration — i.v. infusion over 20-30 min

Toxicity	+ + +	Nausea and vomiting
		Hypocalcaemia
	+ +	Phlebitis
		Pyrexia
		Coagulopathy
		Myelosuppression
		Drowsiness
	+	Hepatic
Monitoring tests		Full blood count, calcium, coagulation screen if indicated
Metabolism and		40% excreted in the urine within 15 hours. Consider dose reduction if renal function impaired
Storage		Powder—2.5 mg vials, refrigerated Solution—only stable for a few minutes
Interactions		Actinomycin, adriamycin

mitomycin C
(Mutomycin)
Group: Antibiotic

Dosage		1.0-1.5 mg/m² daily, till toxicity or 20-25 mg/m² i.v., every 3-6 weeks
Administration		i.v. bolus + N. saline flush
Precautions		May cause severe phlebitis and pain at the site of injection
		Prolonged myelosuppression
Toxicity	+ + +	Myelosuppression (nadir at 3-4 weeks; recovery by 6-8 weeks)
		Phlebitis and pain
	+ +	Nausea and vomiting
		Anorexia
		Mucositis
		Diarrhoea
		Alopecia
Monitoring tests		Full blood count and renal function
Metabolism and excretion		Metabolised primarily in the liver. About 10% excreted unchanged in the urine
Storage		Powder—5 mg vials, room temperature

Storage *cont.*	Solution—only stable for a few minutes

mitotane*
(op-DDD)
Group: Hormonal agent, anti-adrenal

Dosage		1.0-2.5 g q.d.s., continuously
Administration		Orally, 500 mg tablets
Precautions		Steroid replacement if total dose more than 3 g/day
		Discontinue in the event of inter-current infection, trauma, etc.
Toxicity	+ + + +	Nausea and vomiting
		Adrenal insufficiency (ensure adequate replacement)
	+ +	Sedation
Monitoring tests		Urea and electrolytes, lying and standing BP
Metabolism and excretion		Excreted in the urine as metabolites. Urinary metabolites detectable for many months
Storage		Room temperature

mustine
(Mustagen, mechlorethamine, HN_2, nitrogen mustard)
Group: Alkylating agent

Dosage		2-6 mg/m² every 3-4 weeks
		0.2-0.25 mg/ml topically (see section 4.16)
Administration		i.v. bolus into fast running N. saline infusion
		Topically (see section 4.16)
Precautions		Avoid extravasation
		Avoid contact with skin and eyes (wear gloves and goggles when preparing and injecting)
Toxicity	+ + + +	Tissue necrosis if extravasated
		Phlebitis
		Nausea and vomiting
	+ + +	Myelosuppression (nadir at 9-14 days; recovery at 16-20 days)
		Alopecia

Toxicity *cont.*	+	Pulmonary fibrosis
Monitoring tests		Full blood count
Metabolism and excretion		Inactive metabolites excreted in the urine
Storage		Powder—10 mg vials refrigerated
		Solution—only stable for a few minutes

oestrogens
Group: Hormonal agents

Drugs, dosage and administration		stilboestrol (0.1 mg, 0.5 mg, 1 mg, 25 mg, 100 mg tablets)
		breast carcinoma: 10-20 mg/day, orally
		prostatic carcinoma: 1-3 mg/day, orally
		ethinyloestradiol (Lynoral, 0.05 mg, 0.1 mg 1 mg tablets)
		1-3 mg/day, orally, i.m.
		polyestradiol phosphate (Estradurin, 40 mg vial)
		prostatic carcinoma: 40-80 mg every 2-4 weeks i.m.
Precautions		Use with care in patients with heart failure
Metabolism		Liver
Toxicity	+ + + +	Feminisation (e.g. gynaecomastia)
	+ + +	Fluid retention
		Hypertension
		Nausea and vomiting
	+ +	Thrombosis
Storage		See manufacturers' literature for individual drugs

procarbazine
(Natulan)
Group: Miscellaneous

Dosage	In combinations, 100 mg/m² daily × 14, every 4 weeks
Administration	Orally, 50 mg capsule

4.0 Cytotoxic drugs

4.2 Alphabetical list of cytotoxic and hormonal agents

Precautions		Avoid tyramine-containing foods because of weak MAO inhibition
Toxicity	+ + + +	Myelosuppression (mild-to-moderate: nadir at 4 weeks; recovery by 6 weeks)
	+ +	Nausea and vomiting (initially but less as therapy continues)
		Neuropathy
		Rash
	+	Mucositis
		Pulmonary fibrosis
		Encephalopathy
Metabolism and excretion		Liver and renal clearance
Storage		Room temperature
Monitoring tests		Full blood count
Interactions		Tyramine-containing foods, antihistamines, alcohol, hypoglycaemic agents

progestogens
Group: Hormonal agents

Drugs, dosage and administration		medroxyprogesterone acetate (Provera, 100 mg tablets) 200-400 mg/day, orally
		gestronol hexanoate (Depostat, 400 mg amp.) 200-400 mg/week, i.m.
		hydroxyprogesterone hexanoate (Proluton depot, 250 mg and 500 mg syringes) 1 g/week, i.m.
		megestrol acetate* (Megace, 40 mg tabs) 80-320 mg/day, orally
Precautions		Ensure i.m. injections not given i.v. or s.c.
		Reduce dose if liver disease
Toxicity	+ +	Fluid retention
Metabolism		Liver
Storage		See manufacturers' literature for individual drugs

razoxane
(Razoxin, ICRF 159)
Group: Miscellaneous

Dosage		Variable, e.g. 150-500 mg/m² daily, for 3-5 days every 4 weeks or 125 mg b.d., for 3-5 days every week or 750 mg, weekly
Administration		Orally, 125 mg tablets
Precautions		Nil specific
Toxicity	+ + +	Myelosuppression (nadir at 2 weeks; recovery by 3 weeks)
		Alopecia
	+ +	Nausea and vomiting
		Diarrhoea
	+	Mucositis
		Acneiform rash
Monitoring tests		Full blood count
Metabolism and excretion		Liver and renal clearance
Storage		Room temperature, 2 years

semustine*
(Methyl CCNU, MeCCNU)
Group: Nitrosourea

Dosage		125-500 mg/m² every 6-8 weeks
Administration		Orally, 100 mg, 50 mg, 1 mg capsules
Precautions		Give on empty stomach
		Avoid alcohol
		May cause prolonged myelo-suppression
Toxicity	+ + + +	Myelosuppression (nadir at 5-6 weeks; recovery by 6-8 weeks)
	+ + +	Nausea and vomiting (moderate-to-severe at 4-6 hours)
Monitoring tests		Full blood count
Metabolism and excretion		Liver metabolism and renal clearance. Crosses to CSF
Storage		Refrigerated, 3 years

4.2 Alphabetical list of cytotoxic and hormonal agents

streptozotocin
(Streptozocin)
Group: Nitrosourea

Dosage		1.0 to 1.5 g/m² weekly × 4 — repeat at 8 weeks, or 0.5 to 1.0 g/m² daily × 5 — repeat every 4-6 weeks
Administration		i.v. infusion in 100-250 mg 5% dextrose over 10 to 15 min
		i.v. infusion in 500 ml 5% dextrose over 6 hours
		i.v. bolus
Precautions		Avoid extravasation
		Acute hypoglycaemia can be induced by release of insulin from damaged islet cells, especially in treatment of insulinoma
		Ensure adequate hydration
Toxicity	+ + + +	Tissue necrosis
	+ + +	Nausea and vomiting
		Renal failure (may be a transient rise in blood urea, or tubule damage and Fanconi's syndrome)
	+ +	Phlebitis (pain at injection site with too rapid infusion)
		Myelosuppression (mainly anaemia)
		Hypoglycaemia (see above)
	+	Hyperglycaemia (may occur after long-term use)
Metabolism and excretion		Liver metabolism and renal clearance
Storage		Refrigerated, 3 years
Monitoring tests		Full blood count urea and electrolytes, blood and urine glucose
Interactions		Phenytoin

tamoxifen
(Nolvadex)
Group: Hormonal agent, anti-oestrogen

Dosage	10 mg b.d., continuously
Administration	Orally, 10 mg tablets

Precautions		Avoid during pregnancy
Toxicity	+ + +	Menopausal symptoms
	+	Nausea and vomiting
		Thrombocytopenia (transient)
Metabolism and excretion		Probable enterohepatic circulation of metabolites
Storage		Room temperature, avoid light

teniposide*
(VM26)
Group: Epipodophyllotoxin

Dosage		100-130 mg/m², weekly, or 30-60 mg/m² daily × 5, every 3-4 weeks
Administration		i.v. infusion in 250-500 ml N. saline (*not* 5% dextrose) over 30-40 min
Precautions		Avoid extravasation
		Avoid rapid infusion
		Do not dilute in 5% dextrose
Toxicity	+ + + +	Myelosuppression (nadir 3-10 days; recovery 7-14 days)
	+ +	Nausea and vomiting
		Alopecia
		Hypotension (occurs only with rapid infusion)
Storage		Intact vials — room temperature, 4 years
		Solution — 6 hours at room temperature in N. saline
Metabolism and excretion		Mainly excreted in urine

6-thioguanine
(6-TG, 6-thioguanine)
Group: Antimetabolite

Dosage	100 mg/m² orally, twice daily
	100-300 mg/m² i.v. infusion
Administration	Orally, 40 mg tablets
	i.v. bolus in 50-150 ml N. saline + N. saline flush
Precaution	Reduce dose if abnormal liver or renal function

Toxicity	+ + +	Myelosuppression (nadir 10-12 days; recovery 16-18 days)
	+ +	Diarrhoea
		Nausea and vomiting
		Liver toxicity (consider dose reduction if liver function abnormal)
		Renal toxicity (consider dose reduction if abnormal renal function)
Monitoring tests		Full blood count and liver and renal function tests
Metabolism and excretion		Rapidly enters purine pathways. Metabolites excreted primarily via the kidney
Storage		Tablets—room temperature
		Powder—intact vials refrigerated, 4 years
		Solution—refrigerated, 24 hours
Interactions		Does *not* interact with allopurinol

thiotepa
(Triethylenethiophosphoramide, TSPA)
Group: Alkylating agent

Dosage		6 mg/m² i.v. weekly
		intracavitary 20-60 mg
		intrathecally 1-10 mg/m²
Administration		i.v. bolus + N. saline flush
		intracavitary (see section 4.15)
		intrathecally (see section 4.14)
Toxicity	+ + +	Myelosuppression
		Sterility
		Amenorrhoea
	+ +	Nausea and vomiting
		Local pain
Monitoring tests		Full blood count
Metabolism and excretion		85% is excreted in the urine
Storage		Powder—15 mg vials, refrigerated
		Solution—refrigerated, stable for days
Interactions		Neuromuscular blockers

4.0 Cytotoxic drugs

4.2 Alphabetical list of cytotoxic and hormonal agents

treosulfan
(L-threitol, 1,4-dimethane sulfonate)
Group: Alkylating agent

Dosage		1 g daily in divided doses, continuously for 1 month and then alternate months if used as a single agent
Administration		Orally, 250 mg capsules
Toxicity	+ + +	Myelosuppression (nadir after 2-3 weeks of each course)
	+ +	Nausea and vomiting
	+	Abdominal pain
		Skin rash
		Alopecia
		Stomatitis (especially if capsule chewed)
Monitoring tests		Full blood count
Storage		Room temperature

vinblastine
(Velbe)
Group: Vinca alkaloid

Dosage		6-10 mg/m²
Administration		i.v. bolus in 10-20 ml N. saline + flush with N. saline
Precautions		Avoid extravasation
Toxicity	+ + + +	Myelosuppression (moderate-to-severe: nadir at 1 week; recovery 2-3 weeks)
	+ + +	Tissue necrosis
		Neuropathy
		Phlebitis
	+ +	Constipation
		Alopecia
	+	SIADH
		Muscle pain (especially jaw pain)
		Nausea and vomiting
		Mucositis
Monitoring tests		Full blood count
Storage		Dry—refrigerated, away from light
		Solution—refrigerated, away from light, 4 weeks

Metabolism and excretion		Liver and kidney

vincristine
(Oncovin)
Group: Vinca alkaloid

Dosage		Adults: 0.4-1.4 mg/m² (maximum 2 mg or 1.5 mg if age >65 yrs) Children: up to 2 mg/m²
Administration		i.v. bolus in 10-20 ml N. saline + flush with N. saline
Precautions		Avoid extravasation
Toxicity	+ + + +	Neuropathy (may be dose-limiting)
	+ + +	Tissue necrosis
		Alopecia
		Constipation (can be severe)
		Phlebitis
	+ +	Muscle pain (especially jaw pain)
	+	SIADH
		Nausea and vomiting
		Myelosuppression
		Mucositis
		Seizures
Monitoring tests		Full blood count
Storage		Dry—refrigerated, away from light, 6 months Solution—refrigerated, away from light, 2 weeks
Metabolism		Liver and kidney
Interactions		Isoniazid, pyridoxine

vindesine
(Eldisine)
Group: Vinca alkaloid

Dosage		Adults 3-4 mg/m² Children 4-5 mg/m²
Administration		i.v. bolus in 10-20 ml N. saline + flush with N. saline
Precautions		Avoid extravasation
Toxicity	+ + + +	Myelosuppression (moderate-to-severe: nadir at day 3-5; recovery by day 6-8)

Toxicity *cont.*	+ + +	Tissue necrosis
		Neuropathy
		Alopecia
		Phlebitis
	+ +	Constipation
	+	Nausea and vomiting
Storage		Dry—refrigerated, 1-2 years
		Solution—refrigerated, 2 weeks
Metabolism and excretion		Liver and kidney
Monitoring tests		Full blood count

4.3 Toxicity

Listed here, according to body systems, are the more common toxicities associated with cytotoxic drugs. This list is by no means comprehensive but is a guide to those likely to be encountered. If any unexpected toxicity occurs, reference should be made to the manufacturer's literature. Any new suspected toxicity should be reported to the Committee on Safety of Medicines, by yellow card.

The following scale of frequency is used:

| + + + + | inevitable | + + | infrequent |
| + + + | common | + | rare |

This can only be an approximate guide as many toxicities are dose-dependent and, in combination, drugs may be synergistic in producing toxicity.

Cutaneous

Alopecia

+ + + +	Adriamycin, daunorubicin
+ + +	bleomycin, cyclophosphamide, mustine, razoxane, vincristine, vindesine
+ +	etoposide, lomustine, mitomycin, teniposide, vinblastine
+	actinomycin D, fluorouracil, 6-mercaptopurine, methotrexate, treosulphan

Pigmentation

+ + + +	bleomycin
+ + +	Adriamycin, alkylating agents, 5-fluorouracil
+ +	actinomycin D, 5-fluorouracil (especially high dose)
+	hydroxyurea

4.0 Cytotoxic drugs

4.3 Toxicity

Rash (all cytotoxic drugs can be associated with allergic rashes but the most common are given here)

- + + aminoglutethimide
- + + procarbazine
- + azacytidine

Tissue necrosis (on extravasation)

- + + + + actinomycin, Adriamycin, carmustine, daunorubicin, streptozotocin, mustine
- + + + vinblastine, vincristine, vindesine
- + + dacarbazine

Hyperkeratosis

- + + + bleomycin

Nail changes (pigmentation, ridging, onycholysis)

- + + + Adriamycin, bleomycin, cyclophosphamide
- + + 5-fluorouracil, melphalan
- + hydroxyurea

Gastrointestinal

Mucositis

- + + + actinomycin, Adriamycin, daunorubicin, methotrexate (especially high dose)
- + + bleomycin, cytarabine, 5-fluorouracil, lomustine, 6-mercaptopurine, mithramycin
- + hydroxyurea, melphalan, mitomycin, cyclophosphamide, procarbazine, vinblastine, vincristine, razoxane, 6-thioguanine, treosulfan

Nausea & vomiting

- + + + + carmustine, cisplatin, dacarbazine, mitotane, mustine
- + + + actinomycin, Adriamycin, androgens, azacytidine, chlorozotocin, cyclophosphamide, daunorubicin, etoposide (oral), hexamethylmelamine, hydroxyurea, ifosfamide, lomustine, mithramycin, methotrexate (high dose), oestrogens, semustine, streptozotocin
- + + asparaginase, cytarabine, etoposide, 5-fluorouracil, 6-mercaptopurine, melphalan, mitomycin, procarbazine, razoxane, teniposide, 6-thioguanine, thiotepa, treosulfan
- + bleomycin, busulphan, chlorambucil, tamoxifen, vinblastine, vincristine, vindesine

Peptic ulcer
+ +   glucocorticoids

Malabsorption
+   5-fluorouracil, methotrexate

Diarrhoea
+ + +   5-azacytidine, cisplatin
+ +   cytarabine, 5-fluorouracil, methotrexate (especially high
dose) mitomycin, razoxane, 6-thioguanine

Constipation
+ + +   vinblastine, vincristine
+ +   vindesine

Hepatic
+ + +   asparaginase
+ +   androgens, 5-azacytidine, carmustine, 6-mercapto-
purine
+   chlorambucil, methotrexate, mithramycin

Abdominal pain
+ +   vincristine, vinblastine
+   5-fluorouracil, treosulfan

Pulmonary

Lung infiltrates/fibrosis
+ + +   bleomycin (dose-limiting)
+   busulphan, chlorambucil, cyclophosphamide,
lomustine, methotrexate, mustine, procarbazine

Cardiovascular

Phlebitis (at injection site)
+ + + +   actinomycin, Adriamycin, carmustine, mustine,
+ + +   dacarbazine, daunorubicin, mitomycin, vinblastine,
vincristine, vindesine
+ +   5-fluorouracil, ifosfamide, mithramycin, streptozocin
+   bleomycin

Raynaud's phenomenon
+ +   cisplatin/vinblastine/bleomycin in combination

4.0 Cytotoxic drugs

4.3 Toxicity

Cardiomyopathy
+ + + + Adriamycin (if total dose > 450 mg/m², daunorubicin
(if total dose > 600 mg/m²)
+ + cyclophosphamide (high dose)

Hypotension
+ + etoposide, teniposide (avoid rapid infusion)
+ aminoglutethimide, mitotane (if inadequate steroid
replacement) 5-azacytidine

Fluid retention
+ + + progestogens, oestrogens, corticosteroids

Urogenital

Renal failure
+ + + streptozotocin
+ + cisplatin (adequate hydration and avoid aminoglycoside
antibiotics and loop diuretics)
+ + methotrexate (high dose — ensure adequate renal
function and folinic acid rescue; see section 4.10)
+ asparaginase, ifosfamide, 6-thioguanine

Haemorrhagic cystitis
+ + + + ifosfamide (give mesnum; see section 4.12)
+ + + cyclophosphamide (see section 4.12)
+ melphalan

Infertility (see section 4.4)
+ + + alkylating agents, procarbazine

Neuromuscular

Encephalopathy
+ + + asparaginase
+ Adriamycin, 5-azacytidine, hexamethylmelamine,
procarbazine

Cerebral atrophy (see section 4.4)
+ + methotrexate (especially with cranial irradiation)

Seizures
+ + cisplatin
+ vincristine

4.3 Toxicity

Cerebellar syndrome
+   5-fluorouracil

Neuropathy
+ + + +   vincristine
   + + +   vinblastine, vindesine
     + +   cisplatin, hexamethylmelamine, procarbazine

Ototoxicity
   + + +   cisplatin

Sedation
   + + +   aminoglutethimide
     + +   mithramycin, mitotane
      +   ifosfamide

Muscle pain
     + +   vincristine
      +   vinblastine

Rhabdomyolysis
      +   5-azacytidine

Endocrine/metabolic

Adrenal insufficiency
+ + + +   glucocorticoids, mitotane
   + + +   aminoglutethimide

Inappropriate ADH secretion
      +   cyclophosphamide, vinblastine, vincristine

Hypocalcaemia
   + + +   mithramycin
     + +   cisplatin (rarely symptomatic)

Hypomagnesaemia
   + + +   cisplatin (common biochemically, rarely symptomatic)

Hyperglycaemia
   + + +   asparaginase, glucocorticoids
     + +   streptozotocin (long-term)

Hypoglycaemia
     + +   streptozotocin (acute)

4.0 Cytotoxic drugs

4.3 Toxicity

Hypophosphataemia
+ 5-azacytidine

Hypoalbuminaemia
+ asparaginase

Haematological

Marrow depression (Almost all cytotoxic drugs cause some degree of depression, except vincristine, bleomycin and asparaginase. See individual drugs for frequency, severity, and time to recovery.)

Coagulopathy
+ + mithramycin

Hypofibrinogenaemia
+ asparaginase

Ocular

Dry eyes/conjunctivitis
+ 5-fluorouracil, methotrexate

Lacrimation
+ 5-fluorouracil, methotrexate, Adriamycin

Increased intraocular pressure
+ + + corticosteroids

Papillitis
+ cisplatin

Cataract
+ + corticosteroids
+ busulphan

Pyrexia/rigors

+ + + asparaginase, bleomycin
+ + Adriamycin, dacarbazine, mithramycin
+ 5-azacytidine

Second tumours (see section 4.4)

4.4 Long-term problems

When there is a high chance of prolonged survival following chemotherapy, long-term problems become more important. They should
particularly be considered when adjuvant chemotherapy is planned
because, inevitably, a percentage of patients will be receiving
'unnecessary' treatment. In the case of aggressive but chemosensitive tumours (e.g. Hodgkin's disease and testicular teratoma),
complete remission is the first priority and only when a variety of
equally effective regimes have been established, can one afford the
luxury of selecting treatment because of lesser long-term toxicity.

Male sexual function

A number of cytotoxic drugs, in particular the alkylating agents,
cause azoospermia. The duration of this following treatment and
the completeness of recovery depends on the dose and duration of
the treatment. It seems, however, that the majority of men who
have received alkylating agents in combination with other drugs for
Hodgkin's disease for at least 6 courses, are rendered permanently
sterile. Other drugs have less of an effect and there are now
a number of reports of men who have produced children after
receiving cisplatin-vinblastine-bleomycin combination for testicular
teratoma. The testes of prepubertal boys seem to be more resistant
to the effects of cytotoxic drugs and a high proportion will develop
normally and become fertile, provided that treatment is completed
before puberty.

Although there is a theoretical risk of teratogenic effects on germ
cells, this has not in practice proved to be a problem. There is no
increased risk of birth defects in children conceived after chemotherapy is stopped.

Leydig cell function in adults seems to be affected only slightly if at
all and testosterone levels are usually maintained.

Sperm banking should be considered for men receiving chemotherapy with alkylating agents, who might subsequently wish to
father children. However, it has been found that many men with
Hodgkin's disease, especially those with systemic symptoms, have
low sperm counts or inactive spermatozoa, before starting treatment. Similarly, testicular teratoma is often associated with
subfertility and changes in the other testicle. In such cases, sperm
banking is not worthwhile.

4.4 Long-term problems

Impotence is a common problem during chemotherapy but almost always has an emotional and psychological cause. Failure to ejaculate, despite normal potency and orgasm, often occurs in men who have undergone retroperitoneal lymphadenectomy.

Female sexual function

Amenorrhoea is very common in women receiving anticancer drugs, especially alkylating agents. Recovery depends on the dose and duration of chemotherapy, as well as on the age the patient. Menstruation is unlikely to return in women over 25 years old who have received a significant amount of treatment, whereas it usually does in those less than 18 years old. Girls treated before puberty almost all develop normally (for pregnancy and contraception see section 3.10). Hormone replacement should be given to young women who develop amenorrhoea after chemotherapy. There is good evidence for long-term teratogenic effects on germ cells or increased risk of birth defects in children conceived after chemotherapy is stopped.

Growth retardation

Growth retardation can occur in children treated for malignancy. Radiation to epiphyses may cause local changes in skeletal growth. This should be avoided if at all possible by appropriate field planning.

High-dose corticosteroid therapy, such as is given with many chemotherapy regimes for lymphoid malignancy and leukaemia, may retard growth and should be kept to a minimum in children.

Cerebral atrophy

Cerebral atrophy and mild impairment of intellectual function has been noted in children who have received combinations of high-dose and intrathecal methotrexate and cerebral irradiation, in the treatment of leukaemia.

Second tumours

The increasing survival of some groups of patients, following chemotherapy, has been associated with a marked increase in the number of second tumours recorded, some of which may be treatment-related. In animal studies, alkylating agents, some antitumour antibiotics and procarbazine, seem to be the most carcinogenic, whereas antimetabolites seem relatively innocuous in this respect. The most important clinical problem is the development of acute leukaemia (usually undifferentiated or myelogenous), in patients treated successfully for Hodgkin's disease, the incidence being as high as 1% per year in patients who have received *both* radiotherapy and chemotherapy, such as MOPP. Similar second tumours have also been reported, following adjuvant chemotherapy for breast carcinoma and long-term alkylating agent therapy for ovarian carcinoma.

4.5 Interactions of anticancer drugs

These may occur between anticancer drugs or between these drugs and non-cytotoxic agents. Although many interactions have been reported, only relatively few are of serious clinical significance.

Mechanisms of drug interaction

Though some interactions have a unique pharmacological mechanism, most occur in the pharmacokinetic phase, that is, in the absorption, distribution, metabolism and excretion of the drugs.

Absorption

This may be affected by other drugs as well as by food and interruption of normal gastric emptying or intestinal function. Magnesium sulphate may interact with drugs in the gastrointestinal tract and anticholinergics, ganglion blockers, laxatives and antacids, may affect the absorption of drugs given by mouth.

Drug transport and distribution

After absorption, drugs are transported in the plasma. Some are dissolved, whilst others are partly or wholly bound to plasma constituents, including albumin, globulin, erythrocytes and other proteins.

Other drugs which alter this binding may, therefore, interact with anticancer drugs which are bound to plasma constituents. Methotrexate binding to albumin may, for example, be altered by aspirin, which displaces it from the albumin. Other drugs which can affect protein binding include barbiturates, anticoagulants, sulphonamides, phenylbutazone and tranquillisers.

Drug metabolism

Most drugs undergo biochemical transformation and these processes may be interfered with by other drugs.

Drugs may increase enzyme concentrations or activity so that the metabolism of anticancer drugs may be accelerated. Cyclophosphamide is metabolised to its active metabolite by liver microsomes, so that enzyme induction, for instance by phenobarbitone, is a theoretical possibility.

The opposite effect (enzyme inhibition) may also occur and anticancer drug metabolism be slowed. Allopurinol, for example, interferes with 6-mercaptopurine (6-MP) metabolism and increases plasma levels of 6-MP, so that doses must be reduced by at least 50%.

Drug excretion

Some drugs may interfere with the excretion of anticancer drugs, particularly those excreted via the kidney. One example is the effect of urine pH and drugs such as antibiotics on the excretion of methotrexate.

Known interactions

Adverse drug interactions have been poorly studied and some of those described are highly theoretical or very rare. Fig. 4.1 outlines some of the known interactions of antitumour drugs. Those which have been reported clinically are shown in the solid squares.

4.6 Intravenous drug administrations

Many cytotoxic drugs are given intravenously, for several reasons:

1. The drug is not absorbed from the gastrointestinal tract.
2. The drug is too irritant to the gastrointestinal tract.
3. The drug is unstable and may coagulate tissue proteins, if given intramuscularly.
4. Higher drug levels can be obtained.
5. The drug has a narrow therapeutic ratio and so accurate blood levels are important.

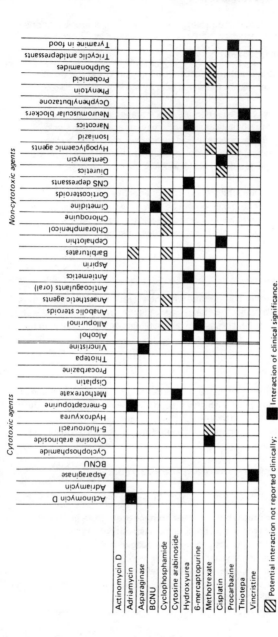

Fig. 4.1. Drug interactions of cytotoxic drugs (adapted from J. Stuart and I. Stockley). Some of these interactions are theoretical and have only been demonstrated in animal models.

Potential interaction not reported clinically; ▨ Interaction of clinical significance.

4.0 Cytotoxic drugs

4.6 Intravenous drug administrations

Because many cytotoxic drugs cause phlebitis and most patients require multiple courses of drugs in addition to blood transfusions and perhaps intravenous fluids and antibiotics, care of veins and techniques of intravenous therapy are very important. Some hospitals have *trained specialist chemotherapy nurses* who give all the treatment. Such nurses not only become expert at intravenous injections but can spend time explaining the details of complex oral regimes and giving the patients advice on preventing and coping with toxicities.

The techniques for setting up the intravenous infusion or injection is the same as for other i.v. treatments but some points are worth emphasising:

1. Find the right vein: use a sphygmomanometer cuff rather than a tourniquet because it gives better control; immerse the patient's arm in hot water for 5-10 min if no veins are easily seen; use veins in the following order of preference : forearm, dorsum of hand, wrist, antecubital fossa; use large-bore veins if possible when an irritant drug is to be given; never use leg or foot veins.
2. Use the right cannula: 21 g or 23 g steel 'butterfly' for bolus or short infusions; plastic cannula for long infusions.
3. Ensure the cannula is in the vein: draw back 1-2 ml of blood; give test injection of 1-2 ml N. saline.
4. Inject slowly: watch for signs of extravasation; ask patient to report pain at injection site; do not force the injection if there is apparent resistance.
5. Flush: follow all injections with a flush of 5-10 ml, of N. saline.

Irritants

The following drugs may cause local irritation of veins:

- Adriamycin
- actinomycin D
- carmustine
- dacarbazine
- daunorubicin
- mitomycin C
- mustine
- vinblastine
- vincristine
- vindesine

These drugs should not be injected directly into veins but into the side arm of a fast-flowing drip. They should be injected slowly (*c*. 5-10 ml/min) and not allowed to 'back up' into the infusion line, giving a high concentration. Watch carefully for extravasation and ask the patient about pain at the injection site.

All these drugs may cause temporary venous spasm, reddening of the skin over the vein or pain along the course of the vein, without extravasating. If any of these occur, stop the injection and allow the saline infusion to run for a minute or so until the symptoms subside. If in any doubt, resite the cannula (see section 4.8).

Alternatives

In patients who are about to have a prolonged course of intravenous treatment, such as adults with acute non-lymphocytic leukaemia or in those with veins already damaged by treatment, long intravenous catheters may be considered. Recently, a number of centres have started to use the 'Hickman' catheter. This is a special catheter introduced into the cephalic vein. The external part of the catheter is 'tunnelled' for a short distance under the skin to reduce the risk of infection. Provided it is carefully cleaned every day and flushed out with heparin, these lines can be kept in for several months and used for:

- all blood taking and transfusions
- all chemotherapy administration
- antibiotic therapy
- hyperalimentation

Patients and their families can usually be taught to care for the line and it can be used in out-patients. It is a useful alternative in patients who are about to embark on a prolonged course of treatment, in whom it is best implanted before treatment starts.

A minor operation is needed to place the catheter. The main complications are infection and thrombosis.

Another approach, less commonly used, is to create an A-V shunt, as used routinely for renal dialysis. Though this may be done successfully before chemotherapy, it often fails if the patient's veins have been damaged by prior treatment and is probably then best avoided.

4.7 Handling injectable anticancer drugs

Until recently, there has been little interest in the potential effects of cytotoxic drugs on those handling them. Many of these drugs have a direct irritant effect on the skin, eyes and mucous membranes.

They can cause local toxic or allergic reactions and there is the potential risk of carcinogenicity and mutagenicity which has not been investigated. Despite a lack of good evidence, there are clearly risks associated with the handling of anticancer drugs and Table 4.1 outlines the possible risks and recommended methods for handling commonly used drugs.

If cytotoxic drugs are spilt, the following procedure has been recommended (only massive spillage is likely to lead to a health hazard):

1. Put on PVC gloves (*not* rubber or polythene, especially when handling mustine).
2. Wear a face mask if there is visible powder.
3. Put the spilled material into a polythene bag.
4. Wipe up remains with a damp cloth.
5. Seal bag and place into a second polythene bag.
6. Label bag with contents and mark danger.
7. Wash contaminated areas with large amounts of water and wash exposed skin with soap and water.
8. Get rid of washing materials in polythene bags as above.
9. Incinerate waste.

4.8 Prevention and treatment of drug extravasation

Despite great care, local tissue reactions occur and account for up to 5% of all adverse effects of anticancer drugs. There are a number of factors which increase the risk of a significant local tissue effect:

1. Some drugs are much more irritant than others. Table 4.2 shows the likely tissue effects of many of the commonly used drugs.
2. The degree of dilution of the drug and amount extravasated.
3. The site of injection. Injections in the antecubital fossa should be avoided, as extravasation is more difficult to detect in this area and slough may expose nerves and tendons, resulting in permanent dysfunction. Extravasation over the back of the hand is also particularly morbid.
4. Old and debilitated patients, often with vascular disease, seem more prone to this toxicity.
5. Patients with venous obstruction (most common SVC obstruction) are at particular risk and it is best to try to avoid using vesicant drugs in these patients.

Table 4.1. Recommended precautions on handling antineoplastic drugs (reproduced from Knowles and Virden 1981, with permission)

Drug	Comment	Effect on skin	Manufacturer's precautions on handling	Action on contamination
Actinomycin D	Not carcinogenic but shown to be teratogenic	Extremely corrosive to soft tissues	Should only be given via tubing of a running i.v. infusion, which should be flushed immediately after administration. All precautions should be taken to avoid spillage on to skin, i.e. gloves and goggles should be worn	Rinse off immediately in running water for 10 min and finally rinse with buffered phosphate solution
Bleomycin	Cytostatic	Poorly absorbed; local toxic or allergic reactions	Wear protective gloves and mask and hold ampoule away from face	Rinse thoroughly with water
Colaspase	Cytostatic; not carcinogenic or teratogenic	Contact with skin should not cause any irritation	No special precautions for handling required	Wash affected area (skin, eyes, etc.) very thoroughly with water
Cisplatin	Carcinogenicity and teratogenicity suspected but not established	Skin reaction to platinum in sensitive patients	Gloves and mask necessary only if spillage occurs	Wash affected area thoroughly with water

Cyclophosphamide	Pro-drug that requires metabolism in liver before it becomes cytotoxic; carcinogenic and teratogenic	Skin irritation is rare	No special precautions for handling	Wash affected area (skin, eyes, etc.) very thoroughly with water
Cytarabine	Teratogenic causes corneal speckling if applied to eyes for several days	Not absorbed through intact skin	No special precautions for handling	Wash off affected area (skin, eyes, etc.) with water
Dacarbazine	Carcinogenic and teratogenic. Caution: avoid extravasation on administration	Irritant; avoid contact with skin and mucous membranes	Wear surgical gloves when reconstituting the drug into solution	Wash off skin with soap and water immediately; irrigate eye with water
Daunorubicin	Carcinogenicity and teratogenicity not established. Caution: avoid extravasation on administration	Irritant; avoid contact with skin and mucous membranes	Wear protective gloves when handling	Contamination should be treated by immediate thorough washing with water or isotonic saline
Doxorubicin	Potential teratogen and carcinogenicity is suspected but not established. Caution: avoid extravasation on administration	Irritant to skin but not absorbed into bloodstream	Protective gloves should be worn	Treat affected part immediately with copious lavage with water or soap and water

Table 4.1. (*cont.*)

Drug	Comment	Effect on skin	Manufacturer's precautions on handling	Action on contamination
5-fluorouracil	Oral administration commonly used with no untoward effects	Minor inflammatory reaction if skin is broken	No special precautions for handling	Flush affected parts with copious amounts of water
Ifosfamide	Cytotoxic only after metabolism in liver; teratogenic and carcinogenic	Irritation to skin and mucous membranes rare	No special precautions for handling	Affected area should be washed thoroughly with water
Melphalan	Carcinogenic	Contact with skin should not cause any irritation	Wear protective gloves and eye protection	Solution of sodium carbonate 3% w/v should be used if spillage occurs
Methotrexate	Teratogenic and carcinogenic	Methotrexate has no vesicant effect on skin but is irritant, and contact with skin should be avoided	Surgical gloves should be worn	If skin is contaminated, wash off with water. Apply a bland cream (e.g. Aqueous Cream *BP*) for any transient stinging. For systemic absorption of significant quantities, give calcium folinate (Leucovorin) cover

Mithramycin	Skin irritation is rare	No special precautions for handling are recommended	Affected area should be washed with water
Mitomycin	Teratogenic and suspected to be carcinogenic. Caution: avoid extravasation on administration	Irritant effect on skin	Protective gloves to be worn	Thorough and immediate washing with large quantities of water. If eye is contaminated, irrigate immediately with large amounts of water
Mustine	Highly toxic	Mustine hydrochloride is a strong vesicant and a strong nasal irritant	Avoid contact with eyes and wear protective gloves	Wash skin with copious amounts of water or sodium bicarbonate 3% w/v or isotonic solution of sodium thiosulphate. If eyes contaminated wash out with large amounts of water and, if available, irrigate with sodium thiosulphate in isotonic solution (2.98% w/v)
Vinblastine	Suspected to be teratogenic. Caution: avoid extravasation on administration	Irritant effect on skin	Protective gloves should be worn when handling this drug	Thorough and immediate washing with large quantities of water. If accidental injection into s.c. tissues occurs, apply

Table 4.1. (*cont.*)

Drug	Comment	Effect on skin	Manufacturer's precautions on handling	Action on contamination
				heparin (Hirudoid) cream to affected area
Vincristine	Suspected to be teratogenic. Caution: avoid extravasation on administration	Irritant effect on skin	Protective gloves should be worn	As above
Vindesine	Suspected to be teratogenic. Caution: avoid extravasation on administration	Irritant effect on skin. Corneal ulceration may result from accidental contamination	Avoid contact with eyes and wear protective gloves	As above

4.0 Cytotoxic drugs

4.8 Prevention and treatment of drug extravasation

6. Previous irradiation to the site of extravasation increases the risk of a severe reaction.
7. Extravasation into an arm whose lymphatic drainage has been impaired (by surgery, radiotherapy or axillary node involvement), also increases the risk of a severe reaction.

Table 4.2. Local toxicity caused by extravasation of anticancer drugs

Drugs commonly causing severe local necrosis (vesicants)	Drugs uncommonly causing local necrosis (irritants or non-vesicants)
Actinomycin D	Asparaginase
Adriamycin	Carmustine
Daunomycin	Cisplatin
Mustine	Cyclophosphamide
Mithramycin	Cytosine
Mitomycin	Arabinoside
Streptozotocin	Etoposide
Vinblastine	5-fluorouracil
Vincristine	Ifosfamide
Vindesine	Methotrexate
	Teniposide

Treatment

There have been no controlled studies that have compared regimes for the treatment of this complication.

Treatment should be started immediately and recommendations include the following:

1. Stop the injection immediately but *do not* remove the needle.
2. Using the needle, withdraw 3-5 ml of blood in an attempt to remove some of the drug.
3. Using a fine (27 gauge) needle on a Tine (TB) syringe, aspirate the subcutaneous tissue to remove as much drug as possible.
4. If an 'antidote' is available (Table 4.3), inject the recommended amount into the bleb.
5. Instil corticosteroids locally, to try to reduce the inflammatory reaction.
6. Remove the needle.
7. Hot compresses or ice packs have been used, though there is no evidence that either is particularly useful.

Table 4.3. Some specific though unproven 'antidotes' recommended for extravasation

Extravasated drug	Antidote	Dose	Mechanism of action
Actinomycin D and Mitomycin C	Sodium thiosulphate 10% or Ascorbic acid injection (50 mg/ml)	4 ml 1 ml	Decreased DNA binding Decreased DNA binding
Daunorubicin and Adriamycin	Sodium bicarbonate 8.4% or Dexamethasone 4 mg/ml	5 ml 1 ml	Decreased DNA binding Decreased inflammation
Mustine and Mithramycin	Sodium thiosulphate (10%) or EDTA (150 mg/ml)	4 ml 1 ml	Rapid alkylation Decreased DNA binding
Vincristine and Vinblastine	Sodium bicarbonate 8.4% or or hyaluronidase	5 ml	Chemical precipitation Increased drug absorption
Carmustine	Sodium bicarbonate 8.4%	5 ml	Chemical deactivation

8. Superficial incisions made into the bleb may be used to release the drug.
9. Hyaluronidase has also been used though its value is unproven.

If tissue necrosis does occur despite these measures, careful debridement followed by an evaluation of the role of plastic surgery is indicated.

4.9 Compatibility of cytotoxic drugs with solvents

Before reconstituting or putting any drug into solution, the compatibility of the drug and solvent should be checked. Table 4.4 shows the compatible solvents for the common anticancer drugs. Other solvents should be avoided as should the practice of mixing drugs in giving sets or infusions. This statement includes solutions used for intravenous feeding. If it is not possible to avoid combinations of drugs in the same solvent, it is advisable to check with the local drug information service whether the proposed combination is compatible.

4.10 Administration of high-dose methotrexate

High-dose methotrexate ($200 \text{ mg}/\text{m}^2$) is potentially dangerous and its therapeutic value unproven. It should *only* be used by those *experienced in medical oncology*.

The toxic effects of very high doses of methotrexate can be prevented if folinic acid 'rescue' is given within 48 hours of treatment. There are numerous regimes for the administration of methotrexate in this fashion but there are several important factors if it is to be done safely:

1. All large effusions should be tapped to prevent drug accumulation.
2. The patient must have normal renal function before treatment.
3. The urine must be alkalinised to prevent crystallinuria.
4. The drugs must be given with and followed by an intravenous infusion.
5. If doses of more than $1 \text{ g}/\text{m}^2$ are used, then plasma methotrexate levels should be monitored.

Table 4.4. Compatibilities of drugs and solvents

Anticancer drug	Compatible solvent for reconstitution or infusion
Actinomycin D	Reconstitute with sterile water for injection *without* preservatives. Compatible with dextrose 5% N. saline
Adriamycin	Reconstitute with sodium chloride 0.9%. Compatible with dextrose 5% in water and N. saline
Asparaginase	i.v. injection—5 ml sterile water or N. saline. i.m. injection—2 ml of N. saline. i.v. infusion given in 0.9% sodium chloride or dextrose 5%
5-azacytidine	Reconstitute in sterile water, i.v. infusion given in lactated Ringer's solution
Bleomycin	Reconstitute with 1-5 ml of sterile water for injection, N. saline or dextrose 5% in water
Carmustine	Reconstitute in 3 ml absolute alcohol, then 27 ml sterile water compatible with dextrose 5% or N. saline
Chlorozotocin	Reconstitute with 5 ml sterile water or 0.9% sodium chloride
Cisplatin	Compatible with solutions containing 0.45-0.9% sodium chloride. Incompatible with solutions containing a low chloride content. The addition of bicarbonate may cause precipitation
Cyclophosphamide	Reconstitute with sterile water for injection or bacteriostatic water for injection (parabens-preserved only). Compatible with dextrose 5%. N. saline
Cytosine arabinoside	Reconstitute with bacteriostatic water for injection containing benzyl alcohol 0.9% and water (*not* for intrathecal injection)

Dacarbazine	Reconstitute with sterile water for injection. Compatible with dextrose 5% and N. saline
Daunorubicin	Reconstitute with and compatible with sterile water for injection, dextrose 5% N. saline
Etoposide	Presented as a non-aqueous solution. Add to 100-300 ml of N. saline — *unstable* in dextrose 5%
5-fluorouracil	Compatible with dextrose 5%
Ifosfamide	Reconstitute in sterile water for injection. Compatible with N. saline
Melphalan	Reconstitute with supplied diluent, compatible with dextrose 5%
Methotrexate	Reconstitute with sterile water for injection or N. saline. Compatible with N. saline, 5% dextrose, dextrose-saline or lactated Ringer's solution
Mithramycin	Reconstitute with water for injection, compatible with dextrose 5%
Mitomycin C	Reconstitute with sterile water for injection. Compatible with dextrose 5% in N. saline
Mustine	Reconstitute with water for injection or N. saline. Compatible with sodium chloride 0.9%
Streptozotocin	Reconstitute with sterile water for injection or N. saline. Compatible with dextrose 5% or N. saline
Teniposide	Presented as a non-aqueous solution — add to at least 300 ml of N. saline or 5% dextrose (watch for precipitation)

Table 4.4. (*cont.*)

Anticancer drug	Compatible solvent for reconstitution or infusion
6-thioguanine	Reconstitute with compatible dextrose 5% and N. saline
Thiotepa	Reconstitute with sterile water for injection. Compatible with dextrose 5%, N. saline, Ringer's solution and lactated Ringer's
Vinblastine	Dilute with N. saline (preserved with phenol or benzyl alcohol) provided. Compatible with dextrose 5% or N. saline
Vincristine	Dilute with bacteriostatic N. saline containing benzyl alcohol provided. Compatible with dextrose 5% and N. saline
Vindesine	Dilute with sodium chloride diluent provided. Compatible with N. saline or 5% dextrose

6. Folinic acid is usually started at 24 hours and the dose and duration of 'rescue' should ideally be dictated by the plasma methotrexate level
7. Renal function should be monitored — a worsening creatinine clearance indicates the need for prolonged rescue.

Alkalinisation of the urine is achieved as follows:

1. Give acetazolamide 250 mg the night before treatment and continue for 2 further days.
2. Give 500 ml 1.4% sodium bicarbonate and 500 ml dextrose-saline, over 2 hours, prior to the methotrexate.
3. Check that the urine pH is greater than 7.0.
4. Infuse methotrexate (1-4 hours) in 500-1000 ml of N. saline if pH is greater than 7.0.
5. Continue intravenous fluids dextrose-saline (with or without potassium) 1 litre/6 hours.
6. Check urine pH hourly — if less than 7.0, give further sodium bicarbonate.

4.11   Prehydration regime for cisplatin

Unless cisplatin is given with a large fluid load, it is nephrotoxic. Because of the need for prolonged intravenous infusion and the nausea and vomiting caused by cisplatin, most patients have to be admitted to hospital for their chemotherapy. Out-patient regimes can be used safely but many patients prefer hospital admission, because of the severe emesis.

In-patient regime

1. Start infusion of dextrose saline with 10 mmol of potassium chloride per litre. Give 500 ml per hour.
2. When urine output is greater than 200 ml/hour, give cisplatin as a bolus or short infusion. The use of mannitol or frusemide is usually not necessary, unless there is evidence of fluid overload.
3. Continue i.v. infusion with N. saline, with or without potassium supplements, as indicated by pre-treatment electrolytes. The infusion should be given at a rate of 250 ml per hour. This infusion should last a minimum of 6 hours or until the patient stops vomiting.

Out-patient regime

1. Start a 2-hour intravenous infusion of 2 l of dextrose-saline, with 10 mmol of kCl/litre.
2. Give frusemide 40 mg at the start of the infusion.
3. After 30 min, give 12.5 g of mannitol i.v.
4. Then give the cisplatin by a bolus.
5. If a brisk diuresis has not been produced by the frusemide, this should be repeated, together with mannitol, until a diuresis of greater than 250 ml is achieved in the 30 min before the cisplatin is given.

4.12   Cystitis related to cyclophosphamide or ifosfamide

A chemical cystitis, characterised by frequency, dysuria and haematuria, is a relatively common problem in patients being treated with cyclophosphamide and is almost universal for those receiving ifosfamide. This cystitis is usually transient and not severe but, if the drugs are continued, severe symptoms can result. Serious persistent haematuria has been reported and total cystectomy has been necessary in a few cases.

Prevention is, therefore, important. The cystitis is caused by metabolic breakdown products (principally acrolein), accumulating at high concentration in the bladder. This can be prevented in two ways:

1. By maintaining a high fluid intake (at least 2 l a day) in an attempt to 'flush' the drug through the bladder in a high volume. Patients receiving ifosfamide, especially in higher doses, should be treated as in-patients and an i.v. infusion maintained for at least 24 hours.
2. By using a sulphydryl-containing compound (mesnum) to inactivate the acrolein.

Mesnum is a new agent that has little tissue penetration and which is rapidly excreted in the urine. It has been used at a dose of up to 8 g/m^2 i.v. and appears to prevent drug-induced cystitis, though clinical experience is still limited. Pharmacokinetic studies do not appear to show any effect of mesnum on the plasma decay curve of ifosfamide. This drug is now commercially available in Britain. For further information on the use of this drug, see Bryant *et al.* (1980).

Other attempted ways of preventing this toxicity have included the use of:

* diuretics
* alkalinisation of the urine
* topical instillation of components containing sulphydryl groups (N-acetyl cysteine), into the bladder

4.13   Oral administration

Most cytotoxic drugs are given by injection, either because they are poorly absorbed from the gastrointestinal tract or because they produce too much local toxicity to be given by mouth. There are, however, a number that can be given orally and some that are formulated for oral use only.

Disadvantages

* the drug may be irritant to the gastric mucosa and induce nausea
* variable absorption
* lower peak levels
* uncertain patient compliance, especially if the drugs have an unpleasant taste or cause nausea

Advantages

* fewer hospital attendances
* fewer venepunctures
* suitable for chronic low-dose administration
* some side-effects (e.g. nausea) may be minimised by dividing out doses

Oral solutions

The following drug solutions, formulated for injection, may be given orally:

* 5-fluorouracil in milk or fruit juice
* etoposide in fruit juice

Special precautions

1. Nausea and local irritation can be minimised by taking drugs on a full stomach.

2. Lomustine and semustine must be taken on an empty stomach, as they are fat soluble and absorption may be impaired.
3. Treosulphan capsules must be swallowed whole and not chewed, as they may cause stomatitis.
4. Patients on procarbazine must avoid tyramine-containing foods (e.g. cheese, red wine, meat extract), because of its weak MAO-inhibitory action.
5. If oral cytotoxic drugs are given for short courses rather than continuously, it is essential to specify clearly the number of days for which they are to be given, on prescriptions and letters to the family practitioner. In general, it is best that these drugs are dispensed only from hospital pharmacies.

4.14 Intrathecal administration

In general, cytotoxic drugs do not cross the intact blood-brain barrier (nitrosoureas and high-dose methotrexate being exceptions) but high CSF levels of certain drugs can be achieved by intrathecal administration. It is believed that such drugs injected into the CSF will circulate throughout the subdural space. This is partly confirmed by tracer studies but intrathecal treatment is often combined with cranial or cranio-spinal irradiation (see section 3.8), because of uncertainty about the efficiency of this circulation.

Indications for intrathecal chemotherapy are:

- proven involvement of the meninges with tumour
- prophylaxis against CNS relapse in acute lymphoblastic leukaemia and some high-risk lymphomas

The following drugs can be given intrathecally:

1. Methotrexate, 5.0-12.5 mg/m², twice weekly, until the CSF is clear of tumour cells. Ensure that the formulation is suitable for intrathecal use and does not contain the preservative parabens or use the patient's own CSF to make up a solution from powder.
2. Cytosine arabinoside, 50 mg/m², twice weekly, until the CSF is clear of tumour cells. Dilute with sterile Ringer's lactate, Elliot's B solution or the patient's own CSF. The diluent provided for i.v. use must *not* be used.
3. Thiotepa, 1-10 mg/m², twice weekly, until the CSF is clear of tumour cells. Dilute in sterile water for injection to a concentration of 1 mg/ml.

4.0 Cytotoxic drugs

4.14 Intrathecal administration

No other drugs can be used safely for intrathecal injection.

Lumbar puncture

1. Standard aseptic lumbar puncture (LP) procedure.
2. Remove a volume of CSF equal to volume to be injected (*c*. 10-15 ml).
3. Send CSF specimens for all relevant diagnostic investigations on the first occasion, and for bacteriology and cytology on all subsequent occasions.
4. Dilute the drug with CSF if necessary.
5. Ensure the needle is still in CSF and inject drug slowly.

Ommaya reservoir

In patients unable to tolerate frequent LPs, or if LP is technically difficult or when it is considered essential to deliver adequate doses of chemotherapy into the ventricles, an Ommaya reservoir with an intraventricular catheter can be implanted subcutaneously in the scalp (Spiers *et al.*, 1978).

The following procedure for drug instillation is used:

1. Keep scalp over reservoir shaved.
2. Aseptic technique.
3. Palpate reservoir and insert 21 g or 23 g needle. Some models have metal cup on the bottom to prevent puncturing both sides of the reservoir.
4. Aspirate suitable volume of CSF.
5. Inject drug.
6. Flush drug through by re-injecting aspirated CSF.

Complications

The following complications may be associated with intrathecal cytotoxic chemotherapy:

1. Fever — if persistent, repeat LP to exclude infection.
2. Nausea and vomiting.
3. Headache and meningism.
4. Chemical arachnoiditis — pleomorphic cell infiltrate in CSF.
5. Marrow depression, especially following methotrexate intrathecally in patients with poor bone marrow reserve.
6. Infection — treat according to bacteriological findings. Infected Ommaya reservoirs should be removed.

7. Paraplegia and encephalopathy have been reported, following
    the use of high doses of methotrexate and cytarabine in
    combination and when the wrong diluents have been used. It
    may also occur when high doses are combined with irradiation.
8. Cerebral atrophy (see section 4.4).

4.15   Intracavitary administration

Intrapleural (see section 3.5)

A number of drugs, both cytotoxic and other, can be used in the
management of recurrent malignant pleural effusion. Pleural irritation and subsequent adhesion is, probably, the mechanism of action
of most of those drugs.

The following drugs can be used:

1. Tetracycline, 1 g—treatment of choice, because of minimal
    local and systemic side-effects.
2. Bleomycin, 30-90 mg—avoid high doses in patients with poor
    performance status or low albumin. May cause collapse and
    hypotension.
3. Thiotepa, 20-60 mg.
4. Mepacrin (quinacrine), 50-100 mg day 1, then 200 mg daily for
    4 days, if tolerated.
5. Mustine—not recommended because of local pain, and marrow
    toxicity.

Technique

1. *Complete* aspiration of the effusion, preferably by tube drainage
    (see p. 76).
2. Dissolve drug in 100-150 ml of N. saline.
3. Instil into pleural cavity.
4. Remove tube or needle.

Intraperitoneal (see section 3.4)

Intraperitoneal instillation of drugs can be used in the management
of recurrent malignant ascites but it is, generally, less successful
than in the management of pleural effusion because:

•   effectiveness depends on the antitumour, rather than the
    irritant effect of the drug

- the tumour may be resistant
- ascites may be multiloculated and the drug may not diffuse throughout the peritoneum

The following may be used:

- bleomycin, 30-90 mg. Avoid high doses in patients with poor performance status or low albumin — may cause collapse, and hypotension
- Thiotepa, 20-60 mg

Technique

1. Drain ascites as completely as possible over 12-24 hours.
2. Dissolve drug in 100-250 mg of N. saline.
3. Instil into peritoneal cavity and clamp off drain.
4. Vary patient's position over 6-8 hours to ensure distribution of drug.
5. Open tube and redrain for maximum of further 12 hours.

Intrapericardial (see also section 3.6)

Although radiotherapy or systemic chemotherapy is the treatment of choice, drugs can be instilled into the pericardial cavity in the management of malignant effusion. The main function of the drugs is as an irritant to obliterate the pericardial space.

The following drugs have been used:

- tetracycline, 500 mg-1 g
- mepacrin, 50-100 mg for 5 days
- thiotepa, 45 mg

4.16   Topical administration

Only 2 cytotoxic drugs are used for topical application to skin lesions:

1. 5-fluorouracil, 5% cream, for treatment of superficial basal cell carcinoma and pre-malignant keratoses.
2. Mustine, 10-50% solution in tap water, for treatment of superficial plaques of mycosis fungoides.

4.0 Cytotoxic drugs

Notes

4.0 Cytotoxic drugs

Notes

4.0 Cytotoxic drugs

Notes

Appendices

Appendices

1   Cancer chemotherapy regimes

This section is included for ease of reference to a number of commonly used regimes. Doctors who are not familiar with them or their indications should refer back to the original references. The short book *Chemotherapy of Cancer*, by S. K. Carter and K. Hellman (1980) is recommended for a fuller discussion classified by site. Space is left at the end of this section for the insertion of specific regimes.

ABVD (Hodgkin's disease)

Adriamycin	25 mg/m^2 i.v., days 1 + 14
Bleomycin	10 mg/m^2 i.v., days 1 + 14
Vinblastine	6 mg/m^2 (max. 10 mg) i.v., days 1 + 14
DTIC	350 mg/m^2 i.v., days 1 + 14

Cycle time 28 days (Bonnadonna *et al.*, 1975)

BACOP (non-Hodgkin's lymphoma)

Bleomycin	4 mg/m^2 i.v., days 15 + 21
Adriamycin	25 mg/m^2 i.v., days 1 + 8
Cyclophosphamide	650 mg/m^2 i.v., days 1 + 8
Vincristine	1.4 mg/m^2 (max. 2 mg), i.v. days 1 + 8
Prednisolone	60 mg/m^2 i.v., oral days 15-28

Cycle time 28 days (Schein *et al.*, 1976)

CAV (small cell carcinoma of the bronchus)

Cyclophosphamide	1000 mg/m^2 i.v.
Adriamycin	40 mg/m^2 i.v.
Vincristine	1 mg/m^2 (max. 2 mg) i.v.

Cycle time 21 days (Greco *et al.*, 1978)

Chl VPP (Hodgkin's disease)

Chlorambucil	6 mg/m^2 orally, days 1-14
Vinblastine	6 mg/m^2 (max. 10 mg) i.v., days 1 + 8
Procarbazine	100 mg/m^2 orally, days 1-14
Prednisolone	40 mg/day orally, days 1-14

Cycle time 28 days (McElwain *et al.*, 1977)

Appendices

1   Cancer chemotherapy regimes

CHOP (non-Hodgkin's lymphoma)

Cyclophosphamide	750 mg/m^2 i.v., day 1
Adriamycin	50 mg/m^2 i.v., day 1
Vincristine	1.4 mg/m^2 (max. 2 mg) i.v., day 1
Prednisolone	100 mg/m^2 orally, days 1-5

Cycle time 21 days (McKelvey *et al.*, 1976)

CMF (breast cancer)

Cyclophosphamide	100 mg/m^2 orally, days 1-14
Methotrexate	40 mg/m^2 i.v., days 1 + 8
5-FU	600 mg/m^2 i.v., days 1 + 8

Cycle time 28 days (Canellos *et al.*, 1978)

CVP (non-Hodgkin's lymphoma)

Cyclophosphamide	400 mg/m^2 orally, days 1-5
Vincristine	1.4 mg/m^2 (max. 2 mg) i.v., day 1
Prednisolone	100 mg/m^2 orally, days 1-5

Cycle time 21 days (Young *et al.*, 1977)

C-MOPP (non-Hodgkin's lymphoma)

Cyclophosphamide	650 mg/m^2 i.v., days 1 + 8
Vincristine	1.4 mg/m^2 (max. 2 mg) i.v., days 1 + 8
Procarbazine	100 mg/m^2 i.v., days 1-14
Prednisolone	40 mg/m^2 i.v., days 1-14

Cycle time 28 days (de Vita *et al.*, 1975)

DAT (acute myeloid leukaemia)

Daunorubicin	50 mg/m^2 i.v., day 1
Cytosine arabinoside	100 mg/m^2 i.v., 12-hourly, days 1-5
6-thioguanine	100 mg/m^2 orally, days 1-5

Cycle time 12-19 days

FAM (gastric carcinoma)

5-FU	600 mg/m^2 i.v., days 1, 8, 29, 36
Adriamycin	30 mg/m^2 i.v., days 1, 29
Mitomycin C	10 mg/m^2 i.v., day 1

Cycle time 56 days (Macdonald *et al.*, 1980)

Appendices

1   Cancer chemotherapy regimes

FRACON (gut sterilisation)

Framycetin	500 mg, 6-hourly
Colistin	1.5 mega units, 6-hourly
Nystatin	500 mg, 12-hourly

(Storring *et al.*, 1977)

MOPP (Hodgkin's disease)

Mustine	6 mg i.v., days 1 + 8
Vincristine	1.4 mg/m^2 (max. 2 mg) i.v., days 1 + 8
Procarbazine	100 mg/m^2 orally, days 1-14
Prednisolone	40 mg/m^2 orally, days 1-14

Cycle time 28 days (de Vita *et al.*, 1970)

PINKEL (acute lymphoblastic leukaemia maintenance)

Methotrexate	20 mg/m^2 i.v., weekly
6-mercaptopurine	50 mg/m^2 orally, daily
Cyclophosphamide	200 mg/m^2 i.v., weekly

Adjust dosage to keep WBC between 2.0 and $3.5 \times 10^9/l$

PVB (testicular teratoma)

Cisplatin	20 mg/m^2/day i.v., days 1-5
Vinblastine	0.15 mg/m^2/day i.v., days 1-2
Bleomycin	30 units i.v., days 2, 9, 16

Cycle time 21 days (Einhorn *et al.*, 1977)

VP (acute lymphoblastic leukaemia)

Vincristine	1.5 mg/m^2 i.v., weekly
Prednisolone	40 mg/m^2 orally, daily

Given for 4-6 weeks

2   Body surface area nomogram

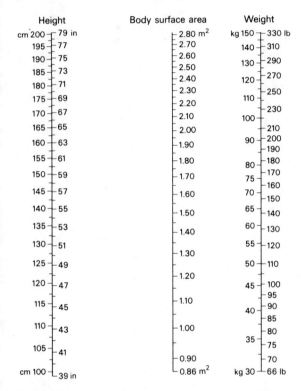

Nomogram for determination of body surface area from height and weight. From the formula of Du Bois and Du Bois (1916)
$$S = W^{0.425} \times H^{0.725} \times 71.84,$$ *or* $\log S = W \times 0.425 + \log H \times 0.725 + 1.8564$, *where S is body surface in cm^2, W is weight in kg and H is height in cm.*

3   Gentamicin dosage nomogram

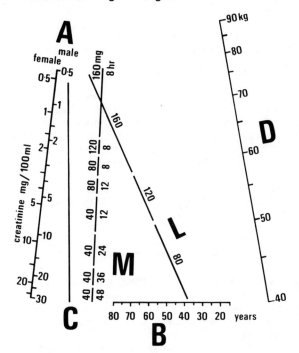

To determine a gentamicin dose schedule Mawer (1974)

Patient not receiving dialysis treatment
1.   Join with a straight line the serum creatinine concentration
     appropriate to the sex on scale A and the age on scale B. Mark
     the point at which the straight line cuts line C.
2.   Join with a straight line the mark on line C and the body weight
     on scale D. Mark the points at which this line cuts the dosage
     lines L and M.
3.   The loading dose (mg) is written against the marked part of line
     L. The maintenance dose (mg) and the appropriate interval
     (hours) between doses are written against the marked part of
     line M.
4.   The nomogram is designed to give serum concentrations of
     gentamicin within the range 3-10 µg/ml, 2 hours after each
     dose. In patients with renal insufficiency, it is still desirable to

perform check assays and to make appropriate dose adjust-
ment.

Example: male, serum creatinine 5.0 mg/100 ml, 45 years, 55 kg;
loading dose 120 mg, maintenance dose 40 mg, interval between
doses 12 hours.

Patient receiving dialysis treatment
1.   When the patient is severely oliguric or anuric do not use the
     serum creatinine and age scales. To determine the dose
     schedule join with a straight line the bottom end of line C and
     the body weight on scale D. Then proceed as in 2 and 3 above.
2.   Peritoneal dialysis. In addition to the dose schedule, add
     gentamicin to the dialysis fluid. A concentration of 5 μg/ml is
     suitable.
3.   Haemodialysis. In addition to the dose schedule, give a booster
     dose after dialysis. Half the loading dose is suitable after a
     10-hour Kiil dialysis.

4   Help agencies in cancer care in the UK

Department of Health and Social Security: grants and attendance
   allowances.
Local authorities: meals on wheels, district nurses, health visitors,
   night nursing; provision of aids (e.g. commodes); social work
   department; domiciliary nursing.
Local societies: provide funds from endowments. The hospital
   social work service will advise.
Marie Curie Foundation Homes, Homes Department, 138 Sloane
   Street, London SW1X 9AY
Hospice care: a number of hospices for terminal care operate in all
   regions.
Red Cross: local Red Cross branches give assistance and provide
   aids.
National Society for Cancer Relief, Michael Sobell House, 30 Dorset
   Square, London NW1
Malcolm Sargent Fund for Children, Chief Administrator,
   56 Redcliffe Square, London SW10
Ileostomy Association of Great Britain and Ireland, 149 Harley
   Street, London W1N 2DE
Mastectomy Association, 1 Colworth Road, Croydon CR0 7AD,
   Surrey
Tenovus Cancer Information Centre, 111 Cathedral Road, Cardiff
   CF1 9PH

Appendices

5 Cancer research organisations

Cancer Research Campaign, 2 Carlton House Terrace, London SW1Y 5AR.

Imperial Cancer Research Fund, Lincoln's Inn Fields, London WC2.

Medical Research Council, 20 Park Crescent, London W1N 4AL.

European Organisation for Research on the Treatment of Cancer, Institut Jules Bordet, Rue Heger, Bordet 1, 1000 Bruxelles, Belgium.

Leukaemia Trials Office, Chester Beatty Research Institute, Fulham Road, London SW3 6JB. Tel: 01-352 8133.

Leukaemia Research Fund, 43 Great Ormond Street, London WC1N 3JJ.

National Cancer Institute, Westwood Building, Room 850, 5333 Westbard Avenue, Bethesda, Washington D.C., USA.

United Kingdom Children's Cancer Study Groups (UKCCSG), The Medical Statistics Department, The Christie Hospital and Holt Radium Institute, Withington, Manchester M20 9BX. Tel: 061-434 3615.

Regional cancer organisations in England and Wales

North Western R.C.O., Department of Social Research, Kinnaird Road, Manchester M20 9BX.

South West Thames R.C.O., Royal Marsden Hospital, Downs Road, Sutton, Surrey.

Yorkshire R.C.O., Cookridge Hospital, Leeds LS16 6QB.

Wessex R.C.O., Royal South Hants Hospital, Southampton SO9 4YE.

6 References and further reading

References

Bonnadonna G. *et al.* (1975) *Cancer* **36**, 252.

Bryant B., Jarman M., Ford M. and Smith I. (1980) *Lancet* **ii**, 657-9.

Canellos G. P. *et al.* (1976) *Cancer* **38**, 1882.

Carbone P. P. *et al.* (1971) *Cancer Res.* **31**, 1860.

Carter S. K. and Hellman K. (1980) *Chemotherapy of Cancer*, New York, John Wiley and Sons.

D'Angio G. J. *et al.* (1976) *Cancer* **38**, 633.

de Vita V. T. *et al.* (1970) *Ann. intern. Med.* **73**, 881.

de Vita V. T. *et al.* (1975) *Lancet* **i**, 248.

Appendices

6   References and further reading

DuBois and DuBois (1916) *Arch. int. Med.* **17**, 863.

Durie B. G. M. and Salmon S. E. (1975) *Cancer* **36**, 842.

Einhorn L. E. and Donohue J. (1977) *Ann. intern. Med.* **87**, 293.

Evans A. E. *et al.* (1971) *Cancer* **27**, 374.

Greco F. A. *et al.* (1971) *Semin. Oncol.* **5**, 323.

Knowles R. S. and Virden J. E. (1981) *Br. med. J.* **281**, 590.

Macdonald J. S. *et al.* (1980) *Ann. intern. Med.* **93**, 533.

Mawer G. E. *et al.* (1974) *Br. J. Clin. Pharm.* **1**, 45.

McElwain T. J. *et al.* (1977) *Br. J. Cancer* **36**, 276.

McKelvey E. M. *et al.* (1976) *Cancer* **38**, 1484.

Peckham M. J. *et al.* (1979) *Lancet* **ii**, 267.

Rai K. R. *et al.* (1975) *Blood* **46**, 219.

Schein P. S. *et al.* (1976) *Ann. intern. Med.* **85**, 417.

Spiers A. S. D. *et al.* (1978) *Scand. J. Haematol.* **20**, 289-96.

Storring R. A. *et al.* (1977) *Lancet* **ii**, 837.

Stuart J. F. B. and Stockley I. H. in Calman K. C., Smyth J. F. and Tattersall M. H. N. (1980) *Basic Principles of Cancer Chemotherapy*, London, Macmillan.

Twycross R. G. in Saunders C. M. (ed) (1978) *The Management of Terminal Disease*, London, Edward Arnold.

Young R. C. *et al.* (1977) *Cancer Treat. Rep.* **61**, 1153.

Further reading

Calman K. C., Smyth J. F. and Tattersall M. H. N. (1980) *Basic Principles of Cancer Chemotherapy*, London, Macmillan.

Clinics in Hematology. The Lymphomas, October 1979, Philadelphia, W. B. Saunders.

de Vita V. T., Hellman S. and Rosenberg S. A. (1982) *Cancer: Principles and Practice of Oncology*, Philadelphia, J. B. Lippincott.

Dorr R. T. and Fritz W. L. (1980) *Cancer Chemotherapy Handbook*, London, Henry Kimpton.

EORTC Cancer Chemotherapy Annual, 1979-81, Amsterdam, Excerpta Medica.

Lokich J. J. (1978) *Primer of Cancer Management*, Boston, G. H. Hall and Co.

Priestman T. J. (1980) *Cancer Chemotherapy - An Introduction*, Farmatalia Carlo Erba Ltd.

Salmon S. E. and Jones S. E. (eds) (1981) *Adjuvant Therapy of Cancer III*, New York, Grune and Stratton.

Saunders C. M. (ed) (1978) *The Management of Terminal Disease*, London, Edward Arnold.

Seminars in Oncology, New York, Grune and Stratton.

UICC (1975) *Cancer in Children*, Berlin, Springer-Verlag.

Wilkes E. (ed) (1982) *The Dying Patient*, Lancaster, MTP Press Ltd.

Yarbro J. W. and Bornstein R. S. (1982) *Oncologic Emergencies*, New York, Grune and Stratton.

7 Books for patients

General reference source for publications

US Department of Health, Education and Welfare, (1980) *Coping with Cancer: an annotated bibliography*, DHEW, Public Health Service, National Cancer Institute, Bethesda, Maryland 20205.

General

Brody J. and Hollets A. (1977) *You Can Fight Cancer and Win*, Times Books Inc., New York NY 10016.

Glucksberg H. and Singer J. (1979) *Cancer Care: a personal guide*, Baltimore, John Hopkins University Press.

Israel L. (1981) *Conquering Cancer*, London, Pelican.

Scott, Sir Ronald Bodley (1980) *Cancer: the facts*, Oxford, Oxford University Press.

US Department of Health and Human Services (1980) *Coping with Cancer*, DHHS, National Cancer Institute, Bethesda, Maryland 20205.

Specific tumours

Baker, Lynn (1978) *You and Leukaemia: a day at a time*, Philadelphia, W. B. Saunders. (Specifically for children.)

Baum, Michael (1981) *Breast Cancer: the facts*, Oxford, Oxford University Press.

Cox B., Carr D. and Lee R. (1977) *Living with Lung Cancer: a reference book for people with lung cancer and their families*, Schmidt Printing Inc., Rochester, MN 55901, USA.

Foulder, Carolyn (1979) *Breast Cancer*, London, Pan Books.

Johnson E. and Miller M. (1975) *A Book for Parents of Children with Leukaemia*, Hawthorn Books Inc., New York NY 10016.

Newman J. (1976) *What Every Woman Should Know About Breast Cancer*, Major Books, Canoga Park, Ca. 91304, USA.

Parker M. (1979) *Children with Cancer: a hand-book for families and helpers*, London, Cassells.

Also see various associations in Appendix 5 for leaflets on specific tumours.

Prevention

Whelan, Elizabeth (1978) *Preventing Cancer: what you can do to cut your risks by up to 50%*, London, Sphere Books.

Talking about cancer

US Department of Health and Human Services (1980) *Taking Time*, DHHS, National Cancer Institute, Bethesda, Maryland 20205.

Nutrition

de Pemberton R. (1982) *Eating Well During Your Treatment*, Mead Johnson, Station Road, Langley, Slough.

8   List of abbreviations

ACTH	Adrenocorticotrophic hormone
ADH	Antidiuretic hormone
AFP	Alpha-fetoprotein
ALT	Alanine aminotransferase
AML	Acute myeloid leukaemia
AST	Aspartate aminotransferase
BP	Blood pressure
CEA	Carcinoembryonic antigen
CMV	Cytomegalovirus
CNS	Central nervous system
CSF	Cerebrospinal fluid
DIC	Disseminated intravascular coagulation
ECG	Electrocardiogram
FBC	Full blood count
HCG	Human chorionic gonadotrophin
5-HIAA	5-hydroxyindole acetic acid
HVA	Homovanillic acid

8   List of abbreviations

IVP	Intravenous pyelogram
JVP	Jugular venous pressure
LFT	Liver function test
LH	Luteinising hormone
LP	Lumbar puncture
MAO	Monoamine oxidase
MSH	Melanocyte-stimulating hormone
MSU	Mid-stream specimen of urine
P.R.	per rectum
PT	Prothrombin time
PTH	Parathyroid hormone
PTT	Partial thromboplastin time
SIADH	Syndrome of inappropriate ADH secretion
SVC	Superior vena cava
TNM	Tumour, modes, metastases
TSH	Thyroid-stimulating hormone
TT	Thrombin time
VMA	Vanilmandelic acid

Appendices

Notes

Appendices

Notes

Index